Ana Maria Cardoso Cepeda

Effects of Radiofrequency on skin wound healing

Ana Maria Cardoso Cepeda

Effects of Radiofrequency on skin wound healing

Digital planigraphy analysis and histological evaluation

ScienciaScripts

Cover image: www.ingimage.com

This book is a translation from the original published under ISBN 978-613-9-63512-2.

Publisher:
Sciencia Scripts
is a trademark of
Dodo Books Indian Ocean Ltd. and OmniScriptum S.R.L publishing group

120 High Road, East Finchley, London, N2 9ED, United Kingdom
Str. Armeneasca 28/1, office 1, Chisinau MD-2012, Republic of Moldova, Europe
Printed at: see last page
ISBN: 978-620-7-66793-2

To my family, my parents Jane and Renato and my siblings Fernanda and Renato Filho, without whom I would not have had the strength and enthusiasm to have completed this stage.

ACKNOWLEDGEMENTS

I would like to thank all those who, with their collaboration, encouraged and motivated me to start and finish this new phase of my academic life:

To God, for life, blessing and protection.

To the Federal University of Paraná, for their availability.

To Professor Dr Antônio Carlos L. Campos, esteemed advisor, for his patience and invaluable scientific collaboration.

To the Coordination for the Improvement of Higher Education Personnel (CAPES) for granting the scholarship throughout the period of this master's programme.

To the secretary of the Postgraduate Department of Surgery at the Federal University of Paraná, Regina Sass, for her guidance and help with the programme's commitments and operating rules.

To my friend Gilian Fernanda Dias Erzinger, a doctoral student in surgical medicine, for her help, motivation and patience at all times during this study.

To my friend and plastic surgeon Priscila Balbinot for her help and motivation at all times during this study.

To my boyfriend Heitor Rodolfo da Silva, for his patience, affection, enthusiasm and understanding during the course of this study.

To Misael G. Barbosa and Álvaro R.G. Machado, for their help during the experimental phase of the research.

To the pathologists Dr Luiz Roberto Kotze and Cleber Rafael Vieira da Costa and to the Pathology Department of Hospital São Lucas for their valuable contribution to the histological analyses.

A word of thanks to everyone.

SUMMARY

Introduction: In view of the number of plastic surgeries in Brazil and the search for better aesthetic-functional results, research is needed to find ways to improve healing and scarring. Objective: To evaluate the effects of three radiofrequency sessions on the healing of rat skin on the 7th and 14th day of healing. Method: Forty-eight male rats were divided into 4 groups (GC7, GR7, GC14 and GR14) according to the group they belonged to (GC: control group; GR: radiofrequency group) and the day of sacrifice (7: 7th day PO; 14: 14th day PO). Under anaesthesia with ketamine 80 mg/kg and xylazine 8 mg/kg, the animals were trichotomised and antiseptically treated with PVPI. The excisional wound was then marked out, measuring 2cm x 2cm (4cm^2) and a 20 blade was used on the lateral edges of the square. The skin segment was dissected. A 6mm metal punch with a cutting blade on its lower edge was also used to make two 0.6cm diameter excisional wounds. After 24 hours, radiofrequency was applied to the dorsal region using Spectra® equipment, directly on the wounds for 7 minutes at a temperature of 38°C. This procedure was carried out three times on alternate days. In the control group, the procedure was carried out with the device switched off. The wounds were photographed at different times post-operatively: the day of surgery, the 1st day post-operatively, the 7th day post-operatively and the 14th day post-operatively. The raw areas were calculated using a specific computer programme. At sacrifice (7th PO day or 14th PO day), the wounds were resected and fixed for later histological analysis using HE. The results were analysed statistically. Results: A larger square wound area was found on the 3rd day after surgery in the radiofrequency group (GR7 3.3cm2 ± 0.7cm2 X GC7 2.4cm2 ± 0.4cm2, p=0.009). The difference between the day of surgery and the day of euthanasia in the GR14 and GC14 was a larger wound on the day of euthanasia in the GR14 compared to the GC14 (GR14 1.9cm2 ± 0.5cm2 X GC14 1.0cm2 ± 0.3cm2, p=0.001). On the 7th and 14th post-operative days, the wounds of the control and experimental groups of all the animals showed different aspects. 90% of the wounds closed in GC14. In GR14, 60% of the rats with punch wounds were re-epithelialised, while 40% remained ulcerated. In GC7, 70% of the punch wounds remained ulcerated and 30% were re-epithelialised. In GR7, 8% of the rats with punch wounds were re-epithelialised and 92% of the rats remained ulcerated. Conclusion: It can be affirmed that radiofrequency has an influence on the inflammatory process, showing that in the rats that received radiofrequency, the square remained ulcerated. Radiofrequency reduces scar contraction in excisional wounds.

Keywords: Radio waves. Healing. Fibroblasts

SUMMARY

CHAPTER 1

INTRODUCTION

Healing after cosmetic surgery is of great interest, given the number of plastic surgeries in Brazil and the search for better aesthetic and functional results. It is necessary to research and improve techniques and solutions for skin repair that is closer to perfection.

Collagen fibres provide tensile strength in the healing phase of tissue repair. Their metabolism consists of a balance between biosynthesis and degradation, which are reabsorbed during growth, remodelling, involution, inflammation and tissue repair. Resorption is initiated by specific collagenases that can digest the fibre's tropocollagen molecules (GUIRRO; GUIRRO, 2007).

Collagen is the most important and abundant structural protein in humans, accounting for around 30 per cent of the total proteins present in the human body. Its primary function is to support the extracellular matrix, i.e. to provide resistance and structural integrity to various tissues and organs, including the dermis. In addition, when immature, collagen is characterised by a large number of young fibroblasts and less dense collagen fibres due to the large amount of water it contains. Over time, collagen matures and thus becomes less cellular and has less water. From then on, the connective tissue progressively matures with greater deposition of mature collagen (GUIRRO; GUIRRO, 2007).

The ability to contract collagen with thermal energy is nothing new in medicine. Thermally induced collagen contraction has been favourably obtained in sports medicine, altering the stretching of ligaments responsible for shoulder instability. This concept of contraction with minimal or no epidermal damage is extremely interesting (ATIYEH, 2009).

Dermato-Functional Physiotherapy can play an important role in facilitating healing, as it has therapeutic resources capable of influencing this process, with Radiofrequency (RF) being the main factor responsible for this facilitation, given its effects of heating the deep tissue while the epidermis remains protected (CARVALHO, 2011).

However, the effect of radiofrequency on healing remains unknown. The aim was therefore to carry out a study on experimental animals to evaluate its use in the healing of cutaneous wounds in rats using digital computerised planigraphy, with macroscopic analysis and histological analysis, and to see if there is an effect on better scar aesthetics.

1.1 OBJECTIVES

The aim of this study is to evaluate the effects of radiofrequency on skin healing in rats on the 7th and 14th day of healing. The specific objectives include:

1- To compare the contraction of the excisional wound analysed 7 and 14 days after the injury, with or without the application of radiofrequency;

2- To evaluate the effect of radiofrequency on the histological pattern of scars using haematoxylin-eosin (HE) staining.

CHAPTER 2

LITERATURE REVIEW

In this section, histological, biochemical and physiological aspects related to the healing process, inflammation and tissue repair will be discussed. The theoretical aspects of radiofrequency will then be discussed.

2.1 TISSUE REPAIR

Inevitably, skin repair results in a scar. Delayed healing wounds with unregulated healing processes, such as hypertrophic scars, keloids, skin contractures and capsular contractures from breast implants or tissue expanders are a problem for surgeons and scientists (TOLAZZI, 2007).

Living organisms have an important self-regenerative capacity. Tissue repair is a dynamic process with successive alternations of anabolic and catabolic reactions triggered by tissue damage. These are cellular and molecular events that interact to restore tissue that has suffered a certain type of damage (MANDELBAUM; DI SANTIS; MANDELBAUM, 2003; RISPOLI, 2006; BALBINO; PEREIRA; CURI, 2005).

The main objective in treating skin wounds is to promote rapid restoration of the lesion, with satisfactory scars from a functional and aesthetic point of view. In the process of repairing surgical wounds, collagen is essential for bonding the edges of the surgical wound. It is also primarily responsible for the mechanical strength of the scar. The synthesis of fibrous protein is the essence of healing (CLARK, 1999; NARESSE et al, 1993).

The tissue repair process is divided into three distinct phases: exudative or inflammatory, proliferative or fibroblastic and maturation or remodelling. Complete tissue repair results from successive alternations of anabolic and catabolic reactions, with macrophages as one of the most important protagonists. In addition to their well-known immune activities, these cells are involved in the catabolic reactions of tissue degradation through the production of proteases and reactive oxygen and nitrogen species, as well as the anabolic reactions of tissue formation through the production of growth factors responsible for recomposing regional cellularity or re-establishing its homeostasis through scar formation (HUPP, 2000; RISPOLI, 2006; BALBINO; PEREIRA; CURI, 2005; VALENTE, 2014).

The simplest skin wound repair is a clean, uninfected surgical incision, approximated by surgical sutures. This type of healing is known as primary union healing or healing by first intention. Wounds with excisions, which create a great deal of tissue and cell loss, are more difficult and present more intense inflammatory reactions, the formation of abundant granulation tissue and extensive collagen deposition that leads to the formation of a substantial scar that generally contracts (ROBBINS; COTRAN, 2010).The main characteristics of each phase of healing are briefly described below.

2.1.1 Inflammatory or exudative phase

The inflammatory phase takes place from the moment of the injury until the fourth or fifth day of its evolution and is characterised by the active participation of numerous cells and factors from the immune system. There is an increase in vascular permeability, chemotaxis of cells from the circulation to the bleeding site that occurs immediately after the tissue injury and the local release of cytokines, which are growth factors, as well as the release of chemical mediators (CAMARGO, 2007; KIRSNER; EAGLSTEIN, 1993).

Neutrophils are the first cells to migrate to the wound site, through the tumour necrosis factor (TNF), they act in the phagocytosis of microorganisms present in the wound and the debridement of damaged tissue through the release of proteolytic enzymes. As the process continues, lymphocytes are the next cells to be attracted to the injury site, releasing chemical mediators called lymphokines, which play a role in fibroblast chemotaxis (WAHL; MC CARTHY, 1978; ORGILL; DEMLING, 1988 apud CAMARGO 2007). According to studies by Folkman (1982 apud CAMARGO, 2007), lymphocytes also release factors that stimulate angiogenesis in healing tissues. This is followed by the attraction and activation of macrophages, which are considered to be the most important regulatory cells in the healing process (CLARK 1976 apud CAMARGO 2007; CAETANO, 2012).

In addition to inflammatory cells and chemical mediators, the inflammatory phase has the glycoprotein fibronectin with an adhesion function, which is synthesised by a variety of cells such as fibroblasts, keratinocytes and endothelial cells. Fibronectin enables fibrin to adhere to collagen and other types of cells, acting as a glue to consolidate the fibrin clot, cells and matrix components. As well as forming this base for the cellular matrix, fibronectin has chemotactic properties and promotes the phagocytosis of foreign bodies and bacteria (MANDELBAUM, DI SANTIS; MANDELBAUM, 2003; RISPOLI, 2006).

Growth factors are also powerful and fundamental in the tissue repair process. PDGF (platelet-derived growth factor) is an important growth factor, acting mainly at the beginning of the inflammatory phase as a chemotactic factor for macrophages, neutrophils and as a mitogenic factor for fibroblasts and smooth muscle cells. Many growth factors secreted by macrophages influence cell proliferation, angiogenesis and extracellular matrix synthesis. TGF-a (Transforming Growth Factor) exerts a strong influence on keratinocyte migration and re-epithelialisation. TGF-pi, **TGF-|32 and TGF-03** strongly stimulate fibroblast and endothelial cell migration, as well as the deposition of extracellular matrix by fibroblasts during the formation of granulation tissue (LI; CHEN; KIRSNER, 2007; CAETANO, 2012).

2.1.2 Proliferative or fibroblastic phase

Three days after the injury, the proliferative phase begins, characterised by intense migration and proliferation of fibroblasts, production of collagen and other extracellular matrix proteins, which contribute to the formation of granulation tissue **and "closure" of the** injury around the fourth day (PHILIPS, 2000) and persist until the 14th day. It is characterised by three processes: angiogenesis, fibroblast proliferation and re-epithelialisation (ORGILL; DEMLING, 1988; HERTIG, 1935 apud CAMARGO, 2007; LANGE, 2014).

The process of wound re-epithelialisation begins immediately after the injury, where the epithelium tries to re-establish its integrity through the migration of keratinocytes and a process known **as "contact inhibition"** (HUPP, 2000; BALBINO; PEREIRA; CURI, 2005; RISPOLI, 2006).

In this phase, macrophages, fibroblasts and blood vessels are present in the granulation tissue at the same time. Soon after the injury, fibroblasts in the wound margins begin to proliferate, reaching their peak on the 7th day after trauma. As soon as they are activated, the fibroblasts undergo phenotypic changes and increase their protein production. Around the 4th day, they migrate to the provisional matrix and start protein synthesis, transforming it into a matrix rich in collagens, proteoglycans and elastin. Some fibroblasts acquire the phenotypic characteristics of myofibroblasts and take part in the scar contraction process. Myofibroblasts have been defined as highly differentiated cells with specialised organelles and characteristics common to muscle fibres and fibroblasts (SCHURCH; SEEMAYER; GABBIANI, 1998; CAMARGO, 2007).

2.1.3 Angiogenesis

In this phase, new blood vessels are formed from those adjacent to the wound in order to provide nutrients and oxygen to the scar tissue, as well as the migration of inflammatory cells to the wound. The tips of these new vessels

are permeable and allow the infiltration of proteins and red blood cells into the interstitial space, explaining the persistence of oedema after the acute phase. The endothelial cells of the microcirculation initiate the angiogenic process, which consists of the activation of these cells, degradation of their basal membrane, cell proliferation, formation of the tubular capillary structure and reconstitution of the basal membrane (SINGER; CLARK, 1999; ROBBINS; COTRAN, 2010; CAETANO, 2012; LANGE, 2014).

The neovessels account for 60 per cent of the repair tissue, hence the name granulation tissue, which derives from the prominence of the vessels in the healing lesion (RISPOLI, 2006).

2.1.4 Maturation or remodelling phase

The maturation phase is the last and longest phase of the healing process. Its duration depends on variables such as age, the individual's nutritional status, the site of the wound, race, age, type of injury and the duration of the inflammatory and proliferative process. By the tenth day, the wound is filled with granulation tissue with a capillary network running through it and the lymphatic network regenerating. The granulation tissue is gradually filled with more collagen fibres and begins to take on the appearance of a fibrotic mass characteristic of a scar. The immature collagen (type III) of the extracellular matrix is gradually replaced by mature collagen (type I) and the number of inflammatory cells and newly formed blood vessels is reduced (ROBBINS, 2001; SIMÕES, 2007; RIBEIRO, 2014).

This process is slow, lasting many months or sometimes years, and even so, a completely mature skin scar has only 70 per cent of the resistance of normal skin. Clinically, it is the most important phase, as the quantity and quality of collagen will determine the mechanical strength of the remodelled tissue (BALBINO; PEREIRA; CURI, 2005; RISPOLI, 2006; CAMARGO, 2007).

2.2 COLLAGEN

Collagen is the most abundant protein in the body and makes up 30 per cent of all proteins in the human body (SINNO, 2012). It is a scleroprotein of fundamental importance in the constitution of the extracellular matrix of connective tissue and provides an extracellular framework for all pluricellular organisms, being responsible for a large part of their physical properties.

The term collagen is generic and can mean different types of chain formation made up basically of glycoproteins. There are around 20 types of alpha chain, which are capable of giving rise to up to 1000 different types of collagen, of which 11 types have already been identified, the best known being type I, II and III. Type I is the main constituent of the skin and is synthesised by fibroblasts, smooth muscle cells and osteoblasts. Smooth muscle cells also produce type III collagen, while type II is produced by chondrocytes. In wounds, the types and quantities of collagen change depending on the stage of the repair process. Fibrillar collagens, type I collagen, form the main portion of connective tissue at repair sites and are essential for tensile strength in healing wounds (KITCHEN, 2003; BRASILEIRO, 2000; GUIRRO, 2002; ROBBINS; COTRAN, 2010).

Type I and III collagens are the most important fibrillar collagens produced by granulation tissue during wound healing. There is a variety in the different tissues and during the phases of granulation tissue formation (ROCHA, 2004; RISPOLI, 2006; SINNO, 2012; RIBEIRO, 2014).

Initially, type III collagen is deposited in the scar tissue and is characterised by being an immature protein. Then, with remodelling, type I emerges, with mature characteristics. In the final phase of scarring, the repair tissue matures, gradually progressing from a cellular and vascularised state to the formation of the scar, with few cells and blood vessels and the end result of a resistant tissue with collagen fibres with a high degree of orientation (CAMARGO, 2007; CAETANO, 2012).

Collagen from granulation tissue is different to collagen from uninjured tissue, as it has greater hydroxylisation and glycosylation, which gives it a larger diameter (FORREST, 1983; CAETANO, 2012).

The deposition of type III collagen in the wound peaks around day 3 and progressively reduces until day 7. The presence of type I collagen increases progressively after day 2 for at least four to five weeks (EHRLICH; KRUMMEL, 1996; VALENTE, 2014).

2.3 RADIO FREQUENCY

2.3.1 History of radiofrequency

The **French physiologist Jaques Arsène D'Arsonval brought about** a revolution in medicinal currents. He invented the galvometer in 1891, when he discovered that the human body could withstand currents with frequencies above 10,000Hz (10KHZ) without many side effects. In 1893, he experimented with a radiofrequency current (500kHz) circulating through a circuit made up of two human volunteers and a 100-watt light bulb, which glowed brightly, while the volunteers claimed to have felt only a warming sensation (GEDDES; SILVA; DEWITT, 1977).

The therapeutic use of RF began in 1920, when electrocautery was introduced by Bovie and Gusting. In 1950, neurosurgeons used it to cause specific lesions in the central nervous system during an operation. In 1960, ablative nodal RF was considered effective and safe for treating cardiac arrhythmias. Ablative RF is also recognised as useful for treating small skin lesions (MATTOS **et al,** 2009).

Radiofrequency therapy uses medium-intensity electric current. The power released increases tissue temperature to levels that favour controllable physiological responses. When used at higher powers and with specific electrodes, it is used to make incisions, destroy or remove organic tissue, known as ablative radiofrequency for medical use (AGNE, 2013).

Radiofrequency has been around for over a century, but in recent years it has gained importance in various procedures, especially in what is known as electrosurgery and in thermal tissue stimulation for therapeutic purposes. Nowadays, interest in non-ablative RF has arisen, especially in the aesthetic field. However, it wasn't until 2008 that the first national device appeared in Brazil, Spectra® ToneDerm® (AGNE, 2009).

2.3.2 What is radiofrequency?

RF is a form of alternating electric current whose frequency ranges from 30,000 Hz to 3,000 MHz. RF's mechanism of action is based on controlled volumetric heating of the deep dermis, while the epidermis is preserved through cooling systems. The immediate heat-induced denaturation of collagen fibres is the mechanism responsible for immediate tissue retraction, while subsequent neocollagenesis is responsible for the later clinical effect (NASCIMENTO et al, 2008; COSTA, 2009).

RF produces electromagnetic currents using radiation. When used as a monopolar therapy, it must be applied between two electrodes. One of them, called the active electrode, releases energy, causing localised thermal phenomena in the tissue, tissue stimulation such as the retraction of fibrous septae and the production of collagen. The other electrode, called the dispersion or contact electrode, is usually a conductive plate with a large contact area. The existence of a dispersive electrode is not a general rule for monopolar mode, as it will depend on the settings of each device. Its function is to establish a current circulation circuit, while at the same time returning energy to the patient over a large area. However, when the current is applied to the tissue, it encounters resistance due to the impedance of the tissue. This resistance to the passage of the electric current produces heat by converting it into thermal energy. The heat is generated due to the natural resistance of the tissue to the movement of electrons within an RF field (Ohm's Law). This resistance, called impedance, generates heat in relation to the amount of current and time. Heat is produced when this inherent resistance of the tissue converts the electric current into thermal energy (AGNE, 2009; ATIYEH 2009; AGNE, 2013; BRAVO, 2013).

2.3.3 Physiological effects caused by radiofrequency.

The passage of RF through the tissue normally produces a series of events that derive from the increase in temperature. There are three main events: 1) ionic vibration: ions are present in all tissues and when they are subjected to radiofrequency they vibrate at the frequency of the radiofrequency, thus generating friction and collision in adjacent tissues, generating an increase in temperature; 2) rotation of dipole molecules: the body's water molecules, despite being neutral, attract opposite charges that convert them into a dipole, thus causing a collision between adjacent tissues; 3) molecular distortion: occurs in electrically neutral molecules and atoms and their movements will be null, due to the fact that they have no electrical charge (BOCK, 2013).

The biological effects of radiofrequency are athermic and thermal, the latter being the most important. The increase in temperature reduces the distensibility of collagen and increases its density, causing collagen denaturation, promoting immediate and effective contraction of its fibres. This thermal injury activates the inflammatory process and the synthesis of collagen by fibroblasts, resulting in altered neocollagenisation in diameter, thickness and periodicity, leading to the reorganisation of collagen fibres and subsequent tissue remodelling. It also produces controlled tissue inflammation, with an immediate increase in interleukin 1-Beta (IL-1b), tumour necrosis factor alpha (TNF-a) and matrix metalloproteinase 13 (MMP-13), the latter being a marker of extracellular matrix breakdown, while levels of matrix metalloproteinase 1 (MMP-1), heat shock protein 47 and 72 (HSP47 and HSP72) and transforming growth factor beta (TGF-b) remain high for two days. Along with tropoelastin, fibrillin and procollagen I and III are stimulated for 28 days after treatment. This thermal damage stimulates wound healing, dermal remodelling and new collagen, elastin and hyaluronic acid formation (BORGES, 2010; BRADLEY, 2011; CARVALHO, 2011; BRAVO, 2013).

2.3.4 Use of radiofrequency in physiotherapy

According to Mattos (2009) non-ablative RF was recently introduced for the treatment of facial and body flaccidity, localised fat, gynoid lipodystrophy and hypertrophic and keloid scars, by means of volumetric heating in the deep dermis and subcutaneous tissue. The first device to reach dermatology produced monopolar radiofrequency. It volumetrically heats the deep tissue, while the epidermis remains protected, through immediate contraction of the collagen, breaking the hydrogen bridges in its molecule. The thermal damage then causes a subepidermal inflammatory reaction, stimulating new collagen synthesis, which gives the skin greater firmness. Atiyeh (2009) states that immediate collagen contraction can be used in aesthetics for rejuvenation, treatment of sagging skin or other signs of ageing on the face or body (ATIYEH, 2000; AGNE, 2013).

2.3.5 Action of radiofrequency on collagen.

Collagen fibres are made up of triple helix protein chains. When heated to the correct temperature, they contract due to the rupture of intra-molecular hydrogen bonds and can generate immediate tissue contraction. Exceeding the heat limit causes the collagen fibres to completely denature. However, too little heat will have no effect. Too much heat can cause cell death and generalised protein denaturation. The RF device, for use in aesthetics, does not need to produce extreme temperatures, as around 5°C above normal tissue levels it is already possible to stimulate the production of new collagen and the retraction of flaccid fibres. Tissue temperatures between 39 and 45°C do not cause any significant damage, only tissue shrinkage, especially of the fibrous septa. Damage begins to be irreversible above 50°C (tissue denaturation), as 57 to 61°C is often cited as the temperature at which collagen shrinks. Coagulation occurs near 70°C. Between 90°C and 100°C the tissue is completely dehydrated. Above 100°C there is a transition to vapour of intra- and extracellular water. And above 150°C, carbonisation or pathological third degree burn occurs. However, for every 5°C decrease in temperature, a 10-fold increase in time is required to achieve a similar amount of collagen contraction. As a result of these tissue responses to RF, it can be seen that there is no single shrinking temperature. The intensity of contraction is determined by a combination of time and temperature. Therefore, it is advisable to constantly monitor the temperature and for this it is necessary to use a special thermometer, usually infrared, whose thermal evaluation is immediate and continuous (AGNE, 2009; ATIYEH, 2009; CEPEDA, 2012; AGNE, 2013).

2.3.6 Indications

The expected results of RF are the contraction of collagen fibres and an increase in skin tone. The main indications for non-ablative RF are: sagging facial and body skin, recent and late fibrosis, scars and adhesions, FEG (Fibroedema gelóide), localised adiposity, oedema, muscle contracture, fibromyalgia, myofascial release, muscle pain. Radiofrequency is indicated in degenerative processes that cause a reduction or delay in metabolism, irrigation and nutrition, and is generally indicated in chronic diseases, to stimulate and cause an increase in vasodilation and irrigation below the treated area, as well as oxygenation and nutrition of the tissues (MATTOS et al, 2009; CARVALHO, 2011; AGNE, 2013).

2.3.7 Contraindications.

The use of radiofrequency is contraindicated in individuals with sensitivity disorders, with the use of intra-organic metals, osteosynthesis, electrical implants, pacemakers, on glands that cause an increase in hormones, pregnant women, in infectious foci, patients ingesting vasodilators or anticoagulants, haemophiliacs and in individuals with febrile processes (CARVALHO, 2011).

2.3.8 Side effects

Temporary erythema is the most common side effect. Blisters can appear mainly in areas over bony prominences. The blisters can develop into scars. Pain and paraesthesia are not common, but can occur (MATTOS et al, 2009).

2.3.9 Human studies

Harth (2010) carried out a clinical study on 30 patients using RF to improve facial ageing and obtained high efficacy, as 86.7% of patients had good results and better results after 3 months, with a reduction of 2 or more degrees on the Fitzpatrick wrinkle scale.

According to the clinical study by Fitzpatrick (2003), cited by Abraham (2007), in which a single session was carried out in the periorbital area in a multicentre study of 86 individuals, measurable elevation of the brow was reported in 62% of cases and clinical improvement of 83% in wrinkles. Also in this vein, Abrahm (2007) reported the Nahm study in which ten patients were treated only on one side of the face with RF and there was a 22.6% reduction in wrinkles compared to the untreated side.

CHAPTER 3

MATERIALS AND METHODS

3.1 RESEARCH ETHICS COMMITTEE

The study was characterised as a controlled quantitative experimental study and was approved by the Research Ethics Committee of the Pontifical Catholic University of Paraná (PUCPR) under registration number 684 on 28 February 2013 (Appendix 1).

3.2 ENVIRONMENT

The experimental procedures were carried out in the laboratories of PUC- PR, Curitiba-PR. The anatomopathological study was carried out at the São Lucas Hospital laboratory in the same city. In order to design this experimental study, a pilot study was carried out at the PUC-PR vivarium in 2012, in conjunction with projects by students Gilian Fernanda Dias Erzinger and Priscilla Balbinott.

3.3 EXPERIMENTAL GROUPS

Forty-eight adult male rats of the species Rattus norvegicus, commonly known as albino Wistar rats, weighing between 300g and 350g, aged ± 3 months, from the PUC-PR Central Bioterium, where the research was carried out, were included. The animals were kept in individual cages, with a stable air-conditioning controlled temperature of 21± 2°C, a 12h light/dark cycle artificially maintained using a foxlux digital timer® with florescent lamps, commercial solid food (Nuvital® Cr1) and water ad libitum throughout the experimental period, totalling 15 days (FIGURE 1).

The animals were weighed and randomly divided into 4 groups of 12 animals, identified by number and group: GC - control group with radiofrequency switched off and GR - radiofrequency group with radiofrequency switched on. They were also classified according to whether they were euthanised on the 7th or 14th postoperative day.

- GC7- control group 7.

- GR7 - radio frequency group 7.
- GC14 - control group 14.
- GR14 - radio frequency group 14.

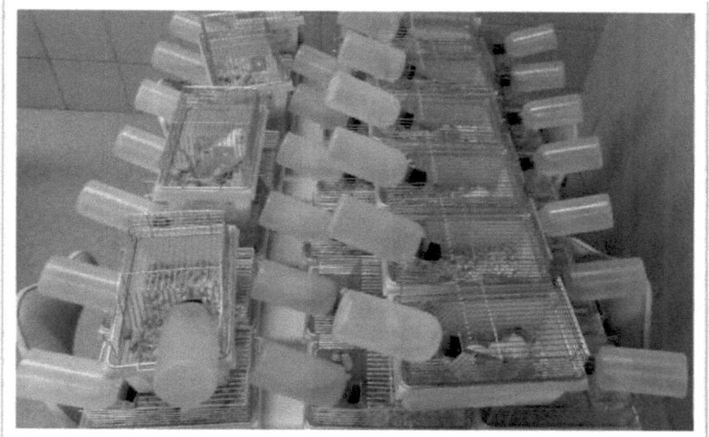

FIGURE 1- ALBINO WISTAR RATS USED IN THE EXPERIMENT.

3.4 EXPERIMENTAL STEPS

The procedures were carried out in compliance with Federal Law No. 11794-08 and the normative document of the Brazilian College of Animal Experimentation (Appendix 2).

3.4.1 Anaesthesia

Firstly, each animal was anaesthetised with ketamine 80 mg/kg and xylazine 8 mg/kg, each anaesthetic being applied intramuscularly to one thigh.

3.4.2 Marking the skin

After anaesthesia, trichotomy and antisepsis with povidine-iodine (PVPI) were performed. The animal was then placed in a prone position with all four limbs extended and the head aligned with the trunk. The animal was marked with a black pen using a 2cm x 2cm plastic mould ($4cm^2$) made by the author (FIGURE 2).

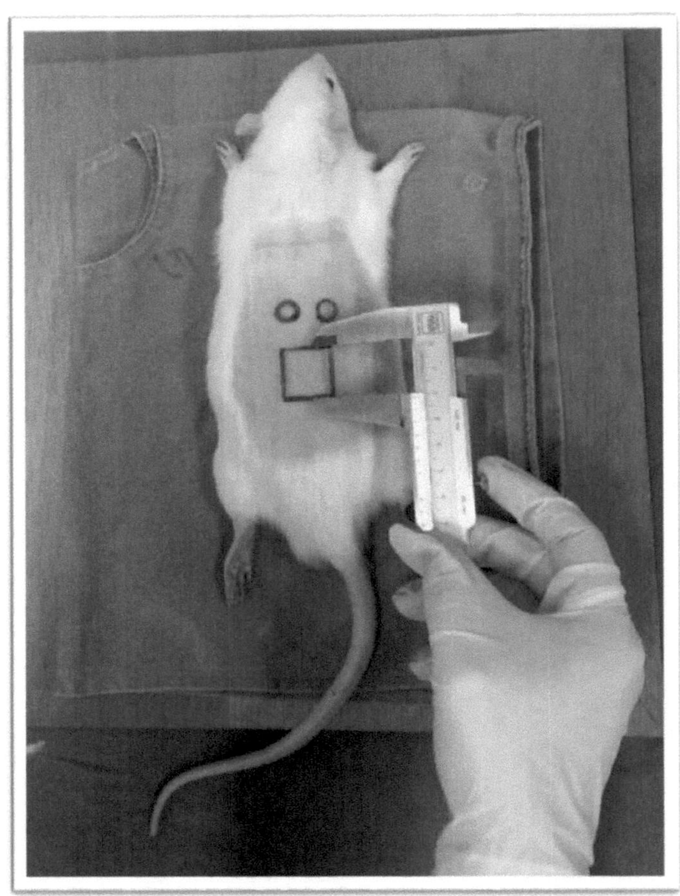

FIGURE 2- PLASTIC MOULD USED TO MARK THE MOUSE SKIN

Markings were made on the back of the rat to make the excision wound and punches (FIGURE 3).

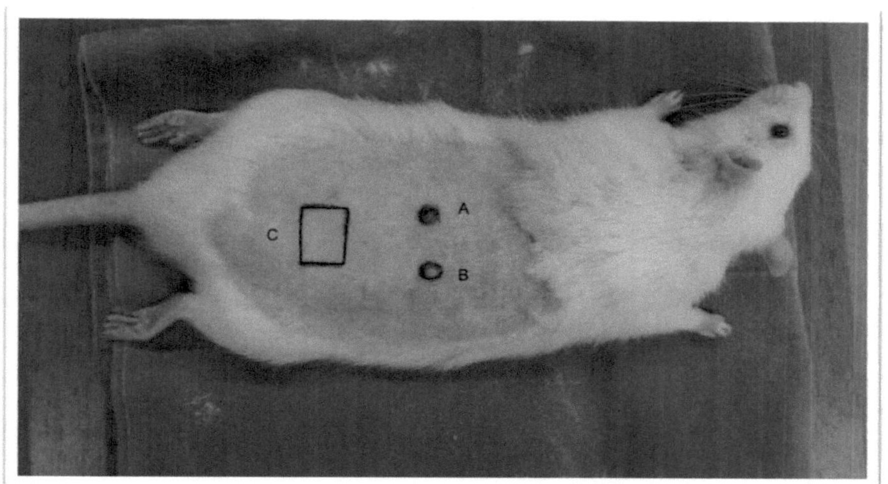

FIGURE 3- MARKING WITH BLACK PEN ON THE MEDIAL BACK AND EXCISIONAL WOUND, DEMARKED BY (A) AND (B) THE REGIONS TO BE PUNCHED, AND (C) THE REGION TO BE SQUARED IN $4cm^2$ WITH THE BISTURI.

3.4.3 Surgical procedure

An incision was made with a 20-blade scalpel along the lateral edges of the demarcated square, dissecting the skin segment. In addition, 2 circular excisional wounds were made. To do this, a 6mm metal punch was used with a cutting blade on its lower edge. This was followed by the removal of two skin fragments until the dorsal muscle fascia was exposed (FIGURE 4).

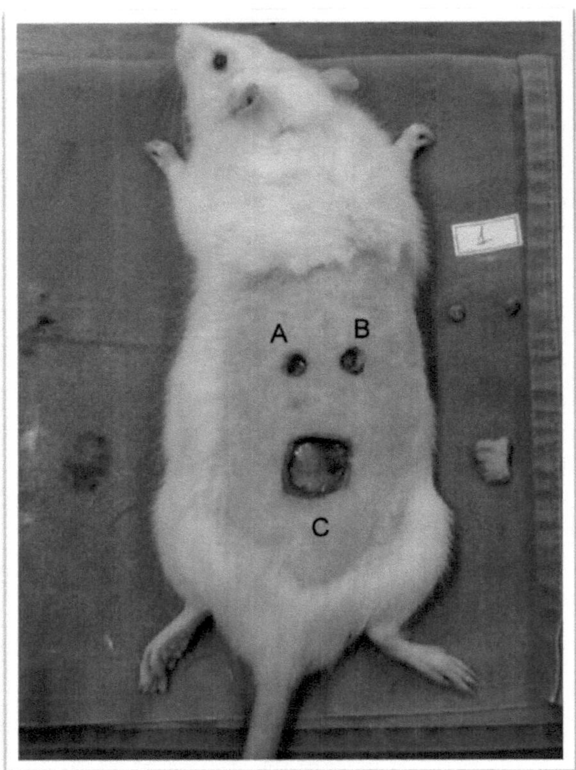

FIGURE 4- REMOVAL OF FRAGMENTS WITH METAL PUNCH AND FRAGMENTS OF 0.6cm DIAMETRE DEMARCATED BY (A) AND (B), AND PERFORMANCE OF THE 4cm WOUND^2 AND DISSECTION OF THE SEGMENT OF SKIN DEMARCATED AS (C).

3.4.4 Post-surgery

During the following 5 days, 5mg/kg of the analgesic dipyrone was administered intramuscularly twice a day to minimise any pain or discomfort the animal might be feeling.

3.5 RADIOFREQUENCY APPLICATION

After 24 hours of injury, the same anaesthesia was repeated, so that during the radiofrequency application with the Spectra® equipment from Tonederm® the rat remained still. The 10 x 5 cm dispersion electrode was placed in the abdominal region to apply the radiofrequency to the dorsal region. The active electrode was applied for 7 minutes, 5 minutes on the dorsal region, and the other

2 minutes were needed to reach the ideal temperature of 38°C. This procedure was repeated three times on alternate days, always with the rats under anaesthesia. Radiofrequency equipment was used with an amplitude of 100 per cent and neutral gel to facilitate gliding. The handle (active electrode) was positioned on the trichotomised skin of the rat's back at a 90° angle and slow rectilinear and circular movements were made over the wound and surrounding skin (FIGURE 5). To do this, the temperature was checked using the infrared thermometer that came with the device, whose measurement is precise and in real time. The thermometer was held at a distance of 10cm and positioned at 90° to the skin. The same procedure was carried out in all groups, except that in the control group the equipment was switched off (FIGURE 6).

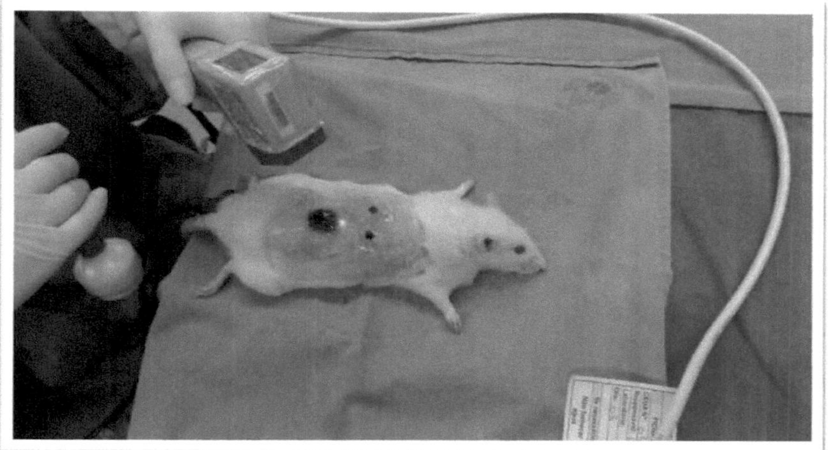

FIGURE 5- MEASURING THE TEMPERATURE WITH THE INFRARED THERMOMETER.

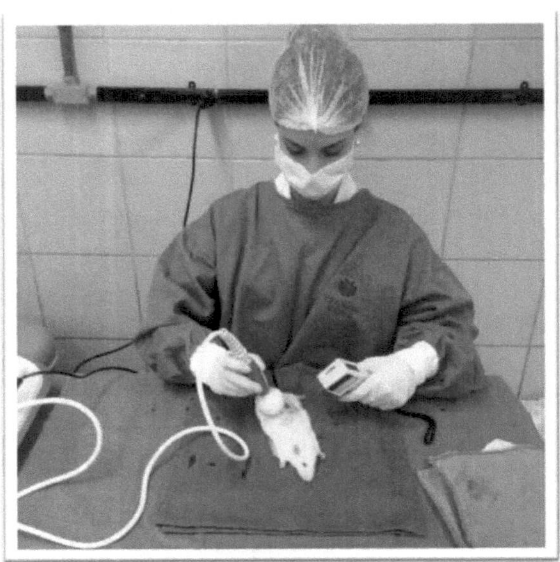

FIGURE 6 - RADIOFREQUENCY APPLIED TO THE BACK OF THE RAT.

3.6 EVALUATION OF SCAR CONTRACTION

The scar contraction of the wound on the back of the rats was compared by computer analysis of standardised digital photos taken 15 cm from the surface of the duly sedated and positioned animal using a tripod.

Photographic documentation was carried out on the day of surgery, on the 1st post-operative day, on the 7th post-operative day and on the 14th post-operative day.

The computerised analysis was carried out using ImageJ® *(National Institutes of Health,* USA), a computerised programme specifically for editing and formatting images (FIGURE 7).

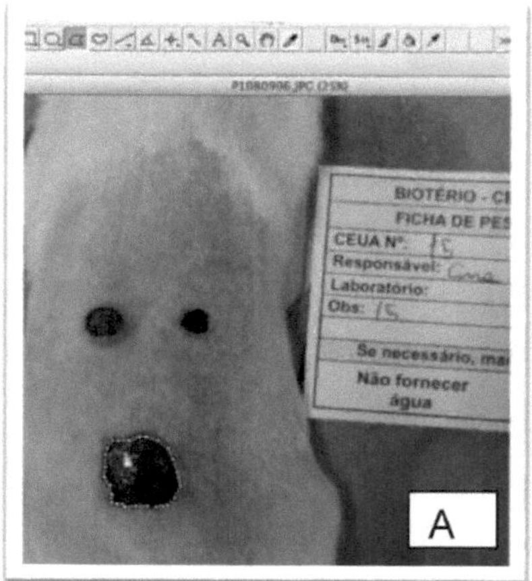

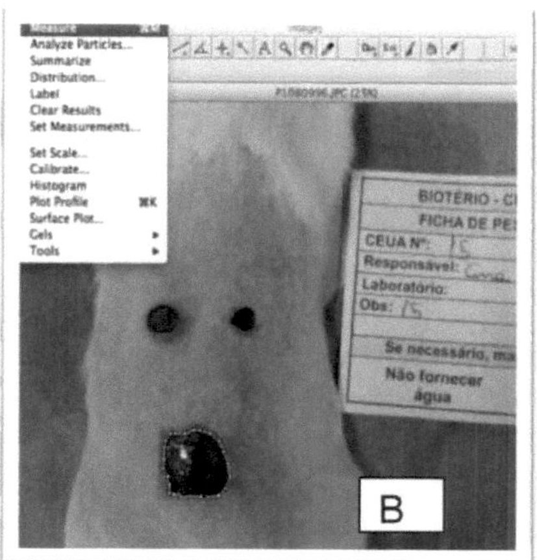

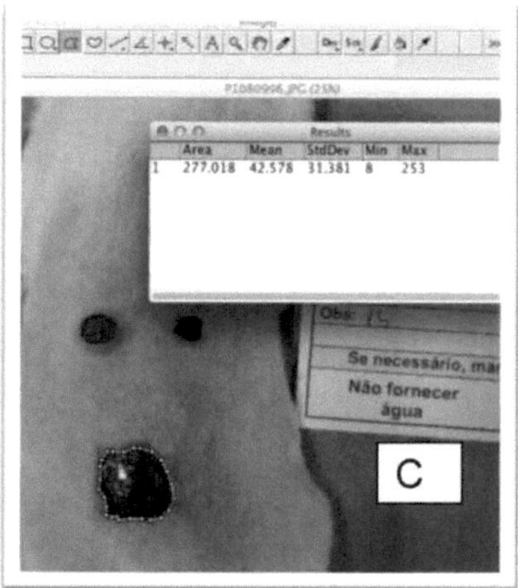

FIGURE 7- TECHNIQUE FOR ASSESSING SCAR CONTRACTION BY COMPUTER ANALYSIS. (A) EXCISIONAL WOUND CONTAINING THE RAW AREA TO BE ANALYSED. (B) USE OF THE TOOL IN THE COMPUTER PROGRAM TO ANALYSE THE AREA (C) RESULT OF THE RAW AREA.

3.7 MAKING THE SAMPLES

The samples were taken on the 7th day in the GC7 and GR7 groups, and after 14 days in the GC14 and GR14 groups. The rats were again given intramuscular anaesthesia and the skin samples from the region were surgically removed and stored in vials with a 10% formaldehyde solution. After this procedure, the animals were euthanised in a chamber with 70% CO_2 saturation. The tissue samples immersed in 10% formaldehyde were sent to the PUC laboratory for histological analysis.

3.8 HISTOLOGICAL ANALYSIS

The fixed samples were cleaved, placed in histological cassettes and processed in an autotechnician for paraffin embedding. The samples were embedded, cut on a microtome at 3|jm, stained using the Haematoxylin-Eosin (HE) method and mounted.

The microscopic analysis using an Olympus optical microscope model CX31® was carried out by a pathologist, without knowing which group the rat belonged to. This made it possible to semi-quantitatively assess the inflammatory cell component, the cellular elements of chronic and acute inflammation, fibroblast repair and proliferation, which were quantified as described in TABLE 1. The re-epithelialisation of the punches was analysed according to TABLE 2.

TABLE 1- PARAMETERS ANALYSED BY THE HE METHOD SOURCE: JUNQUEIRA (2004)

GRAU	**Cellular inflammatory component**	**Cellular elements of chronic inflammation: lymphocytes**	**Cellular elements of acute inflammation: neutrophils**	**Repair: macrophages, granulomas**	**Fibroblast proliferation**
0	Absence of cellular elements	Absence of lymp hocytesor plasma cells	Absence of neutrophils, capillary congestion	No evidence of repair	Young fibroblasts are not observed
1	Inflammatory cells in small numbers(near vessels)	Small number of lymphocytes and/or plasma cells	Small number of neutrophils in the dermis	Small numbers of macrophages	Fibroblasts are seen in areas of loose collagen
2	Inflammatory cells in moderate numbers, sparse	Moderate number of lymphocytes and/or plasma cells	Moderate number of neutrophils	Macrophages in moderate quantity	Fibroblasts are easily seen, collagen matrix visible
3	Inflammatory cells in moderate numbers, clustered s	Numerous lymphocytes/ plasma cells	Neutrophilic exudate	Macrophages in mod.num, without specific arrangement.	Easily observed fibroblasts, collagen matrix and capillary proliferation
4	Numerous inflammatory cells	Numerous lymph nodes, lymphoids, lymphocytic crowns	Neutrophilic exudate, abscesses	Macrophages arranged in granulomas	Fibroblasts are numerous, collagen matrix present, capillary proliferation

As the parameters used in the HE assessment were subjective, they were graded from 0, the smallest number of cells found, to 4 containing numerous cells, in order to transform this data into numerical values and allow statistical analysis.

CHART 2 - METHOD USED TO ANALYSE THE RE-EPITHELIALISATION OF PUNCH INJURIES.

	Reepithelialisation
+	Intact epidermis
-	Epidermal continuity solution associated with inflammation and/or crusts (ulceration)

3.9 STATISTICAL ANALYSIS

All the data was tabulated in a **Microsoft Office Excel** spreadsheet® and the results of the quantitative variables were described by mean and standard deviation. Student's t-test for independent samples was used to compare the two groups in terms of the area assessed at the time of surgery. This comparison for the area assessments on day 1, day 3 and the day of euthanasia and for the differences in area in relation to the time of surgery was made using the analysis of covariance (ANCOVA) model including the area at surgery as a co-variable. The analysis of variance model with repeated measures (ANOVA) and the LSD (least significant difference) test for multiple comparisons were used to compare the four assessment times in relation to area. The Mann-Whitney non-parametric test was used to compare two groups in relation to the HE variables. With regard to the ulceration variable, the groups were compared using 1-way ANOVA with Turkey's post-test. Values of $p<0.05$ indicated statistical significance. The data was analysed using IBM SPSS v.20 and Graph pad prism 5.0.

CHAPTER 4

RESULTS

During data collection, the number of rats decreased from 48 to 43, 5 rats died during the radiofrequency procedures and were withdrawn from the research.

4.1 COMPARISONS OF THE GROUPS IN RELATION TO THE ASSESSMENT OF THE WOUND AREA.

The evolution of the reduction in the lesion area at each of the times of the experiment, analysed by digital planigraphy, is shown in the graphs below (GRAPHS 1,2).

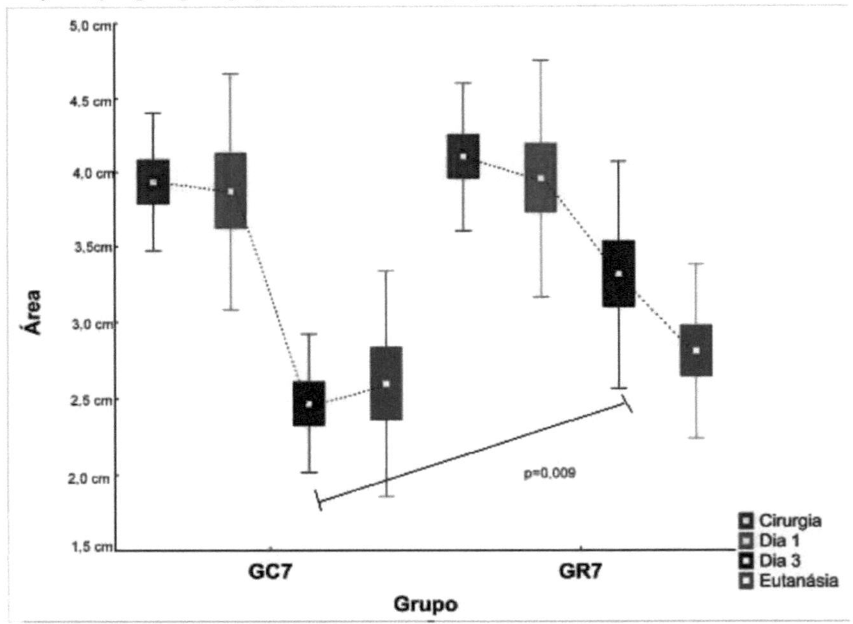

GRAPH 1- COMPARISON OF GROUPS GR7 AND GC7 IN RELATION TO AREA ASSESSMENTS AT SURGERY, 1 DAY, 3 DAYS AND EUTHANASIA.

It can be seen that the average area on day 3 in the GR7 group is greater than the area in the GC7 group (GR7 $3.3cm^2 \pm 0.7cm^2$ X GC7 $2.4cm^2 \pm 0.4cm^2$, $p=0.009$). The graph above shows that in the GR7 group the area gradually decreases over time. In the GC7 group, there was a significant decrease from the 1st to the 3rd day.

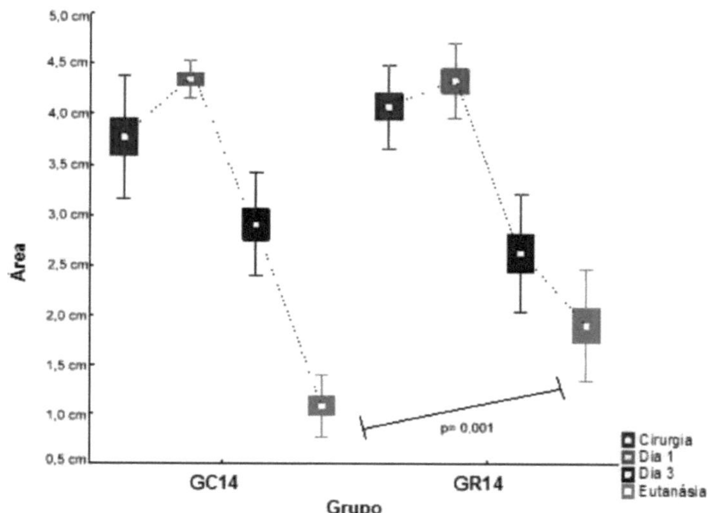

GRAPH 2- COMPARISON OF THE GR14 AND GC14 GROUPS IN RELATION TO AREA ASSESSMENTS AT SURGERY, 1 DAY, 3 DAYS AND EUTHANASIA.

The GR14 found a larger area than the GC14 on the day of euthanasia, with a significant difference between the groups (GR14 $1.9cm^2 \pm 0.5cm^2$ X GC14 $1.0cm^2 \pm 0.3cm^2$, p=0.001) It can be seen in the graph above that both groups show a decline in area on the 3rd day, however in the GR14 group there is a smaller decrease in wound area on the day of euthanasia than in the GC14 group.

4.2 MACROSCOPIC ANALYSIS

On the 7th and 14th post-operative days, the wounds of the control and experimental groups of all the animals showed different aspects. Ninety per cent of the wounds in GC14 were closed, while 10 per cent remained ulcerated. In GR14, 60% of the rats with punch wounds were re-epithelialised while 40% remained ulcerated. Showing a significant difference between GR14 and GC14 with p=0.018. In GC7, 70% of the punch wounds remained ulcerated and 30% were re-epithelialised. In GR7, 8% of the rats with punch wounds were re-epithelialised and 92% of the rats remained ulcerated (TABLE 1).

TABLE 1- COMPARISON OF THE CONTROL AND RADIOFREQUENCY GROUPS AT DAY 7 AND 14 IN RELATION TO THE VARIABLE ULCERATION.

ULCERATION	GC7	GR7	GC14	GR14
n	10	12	11	10
PRESENT(%)	70	92	10	40

ABSENT(%)	30	8*	90	60**

*p=0,500
**p=0,018

Statistical test: 1-way ANOVA with Turkey post-test

Figures 8 and 9 show an example of the evolution in detail of the *punch* and square wounds, on the days of surgery, 1st day P.O., 3rd day P.O. and euthanasia on the 7th day P.O. of GC7.

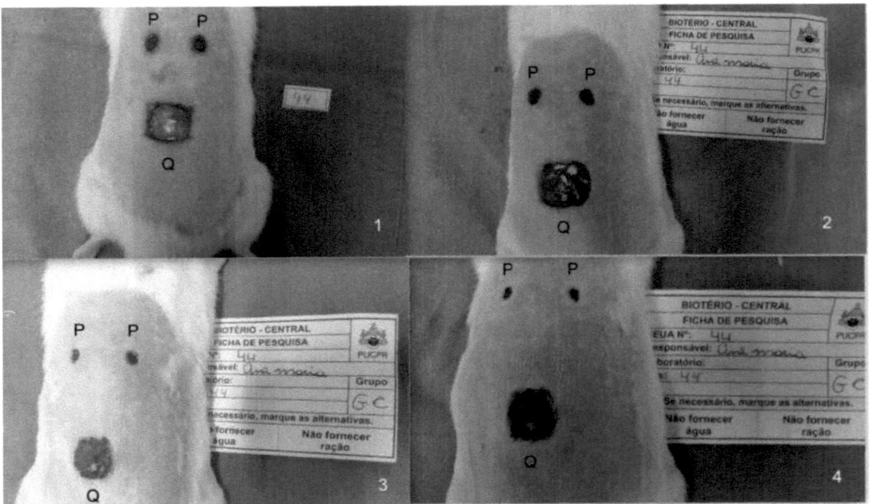

FIGURA 8: EXAMPLE OF PUNCH AND SQUARE WOUNDS REPRESENTED BY P (PUNCH) Q (SQUARE) OF GC7 ON DAY OF SURGERY (1), 1ST DAY P.O (2), 3RD DAY P.O (3) AND EUTHANASIA 7TH DAY P.O (4).

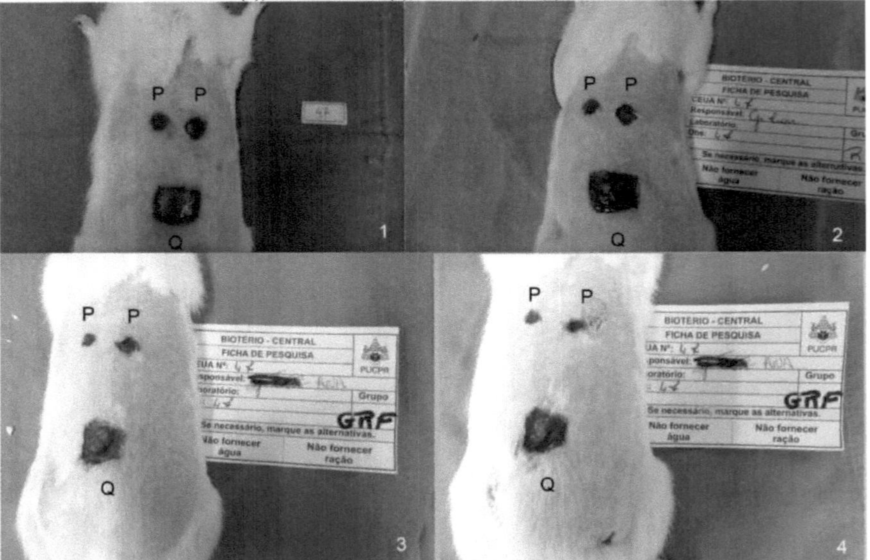

FIGURA 9: EXAMPLE OF PUNCH AND SQUARE WOUNDS REPRESENTED BY P (PUNCH) Q (SQUARE)

FROM GR7 ON DAY OF SURGERY (1), 1ST DAY P.O (2), 3RD DAY P.O (3) AND EUTHANASIA 7TH DAY P.O (4).

An example is shown in Figures 10 and 11, in the punch and square wounds of GC14 performed on the day of surgery, 1st day P.O., 3rd day P.O. and euthanasia on the 14th day P.O.

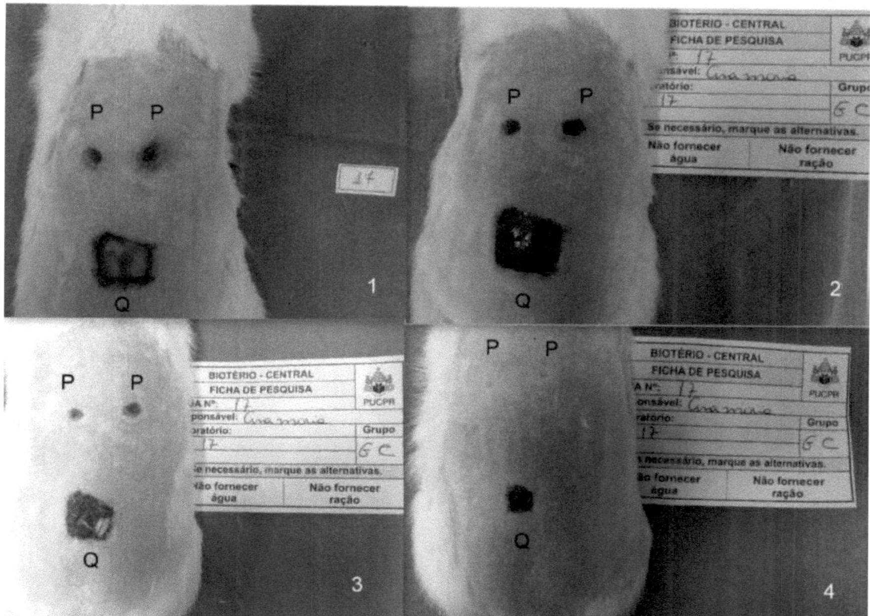

FIGURA 10: EXAMPLE OF PUNCH AND SQUARE WOUNDS REPRESENTED BY P (PUNCH) Q (SQUARE) OF GC14 FROM DAY OF SURGERY (1), 1ST DAY P.O (2), 3RD DAY P.O (3) AND EUTHANASIA 14TH DAY P.O (4).

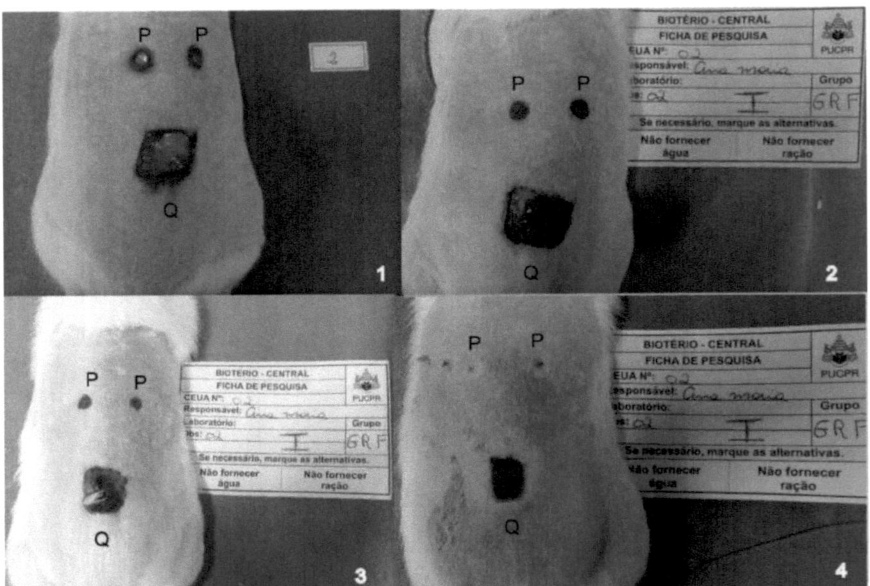

FIGURA 11: EXAMPLE OF PUNCH AND SQUARE WOUNDS REPRESENTED BY P (PUNCH) Q (SQUARE) FROM GR14 ON DAY OF SURGERY (1), DAY 1 P.O (2), DAY 3 P.O (3) AND EUTHANASIA DAY 14 P.O (4).

The detail in figure 12 shows significant macroscopic changes.

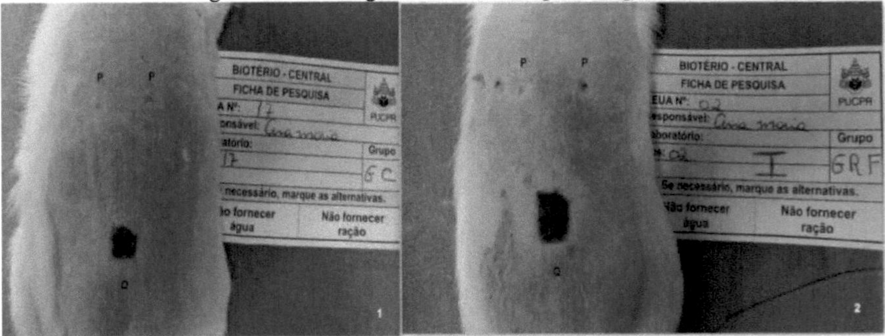

FIGURA 12: IN FIGURE 1, WE CAN SEE THAT IN GC14 THE PUNCHES ARE CLOSED, WHILE IN FIGURE 2 IN GR14 THE PUNCHES ARE MORE OPEN. WE CAN ALSO SEE THAT IN GR14 THE SQUARE IS LARGER WHEN COMPARED TO THE SQUARE IN GC14.

4.3 COMPARISON OF THE GC AND GR GROUPS IN RELATION TO HEALTH VARIABLES

Only in GR7, in the evaluation of chronic inflammation cells, was there difference between the groups (GR7 1.9 ± 0.7 X GC7 2.5 ± 0.5, p= 0.05) (TABLE 2).

TABLE 2 - COMPARISON OF GROUPS GC7 AND GR7 IN RELATION TO THE VARIABLES HE, INFLAMMATION, CHRONIC INFLAMMATION, ACUTE INFLAMMATION, FIBROBLAST PROLIFERATION.

QUADRADO-Q - 7 days

Variable	Group	N	Media± dp	p-value* (GC x GR)
Q-Inflammation	GC7	10	2,8±0,4	
	GR7	12	2,6±0,5	0,381
Q-Chronic inflammation	GC7	10	2,5±0,5	
	GR7	12	1,9±0,7	0,050
Q-Acute inflammation	GC7	10	2,0±0,5	
	GR7	12	2,5±1,1	0,539
Q-Proliferation Fibroblastic	GC7	10	2,9±0,3	
	GR7	12	2,7±0,5	0,381
Q-Repair	GC7	10	1,5±0,7	
	GR7	12	1,6±1,0	0,872

*Student's t-test; **p** < 0.05

The GR14 showed an increase in acute inflammation cells (GR14 3.2 ± 0.9 x GC14 1.5 ± 0.9, p=0.001) and for the inflammation variable, the GR14 also showed a higher number of cells (GR14 3.2 ± 0.6 x GC14 2.4 ± 0.5, p=0.01) (TABLE 3).

TABLE 3 - COMPARISON OF THE GC14 AND GR14 GROUPS IN RELATION TO THE VARIABLES HE, INFLAMMATION, CHRONIC INFLAMMATION, ACUTE INFLAMMATION, FIBROBLAST PROLIFERATION.

QUADRADO-Q - 14 days

Variable	Group	N	Mean ± SD	p-value* (GC x GR)
Q-Inflammation	GC14	11	2,4±0,5	
	GR14	10	3,2±0,6	0,010
Q-Chronic inflammation	GC14	11	2,2±0,4	
	GR14	10	1,9±0,6	0,349
Q-Acute inflammation	GC14	11	1,5±0,9	
	GR14	10	3,2±0,9	0,001
Q-Fibroblast proliferation	GC14	11	2,5±0,5	
	GR14	10	2,4±0,8	0,918
Q-Repair	GC14	11	2,4±1,3	
	GR14	10	1,3±0,7	0,061

*Student's t-test; **p** <0.05

4.4 COMPARISON OF THE SQUARE WOUNDS ON THE EVALUATION DAYS, WITHIN THE GC AND GR GROUPS, IN RELATION TO THE HE VARIABLES.

The mean inflammation was similar in GR7 and GC7 (GR7 2.6 ± 0.5 X GC7 2.8 ± 0.4, p=0.3), which shows inflammatory cells in moderate numbers and sparse. The higher mean in GR14 compared to GC14 (GR14 3.2 ± 0.6 X GC14 2.4 ± 0.5, p=0.01) showed inflammatory cells in moderate numbers and clusters of cells. (GRAPH 3)

Chronic inflammation remained the same in GR7 and GR14 (GR7 1.9 ± 0.7 X GR14 1.9 ± 6, p=0.82), showing a small number of lymphocytes and/or plasma cells on the different days of euthanasia, while in GC7 and GC14 these cellular elements of chronic inflammation showed a moderate number of lymphocytes and/or plasma cells (GC7 2.5 ± 0.5 X GC14 2.2 ± 0.4, p=0.22).

When analysing the cellular elements of acute inflammation, the GR7 had a similar number of cells to the GC7 (GR7 2.5 ± 1.1 X GC7 2.0 ± 0.5, p=0.53) and a higher number of neutrophils (acute inflammation) in the GR14 x GC14 (GR14 3.2 ± 0.9 X GC14 1.5 ± 0.9, p=0.001).

Fibroblast proliferation was similar between the GR7 and GC7 groups (GR7 2.7 ± 0.5 X GC7 2.9 ± 0.3, p=0.38) with easily observed fibroblasts, collagen matrix and capillary proliferation. GR14 and GC14 were also similar, with easily observed fibroblasts and visible collagen matrix (GR14 2.4 ± 0.8 X GC14 2.5 ± 0.5, p=0.91).

The repair showed macrophages in small numbers and was similar in the GR7 and GC7 groups (GR7 1.6 ± 1.0 X GC7 1.5 ± 0.7, p=0.87), but GR14 showed a tendency towards fewer macrophages compared to GC14, with macrophages in small numbers, while in GC14 the presence of macrophages was moderate, (GR14 1.3 ± 0.7 X GC14 2.4 ± 1.3, p=0.06).

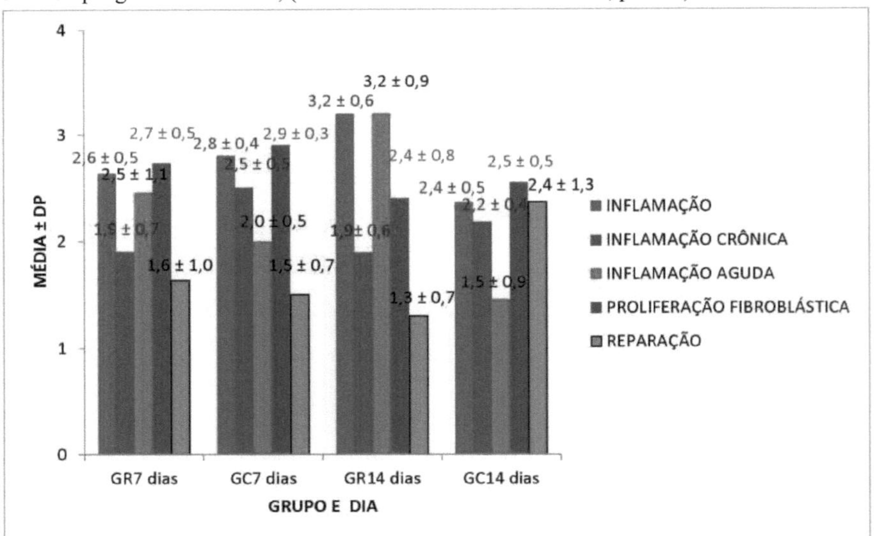

GRAPH 3- COMPARISON OF THE ANALYSES MADE BY HE IN RELATION TO INFLAMMATION, CHRONIC INFLAMMATION, ACUTE INFLAMMATION, FIBROBLAST PROLIFERATION AND REPAIR IN THE CONTROL GROUP GC AND RADIOFREQUENCY GROUP GR ON THE 7TH DAY OF EUTHANASIA AND THE 14TH DAY OF EUTHANASIA.

CHAPTER 5

DISCUSSION

The Wistar rat is commonly used as an experimental model for the study of scarring, as it is a small animal, resistant to infections, easy to acquire and standardise in terms of age, weight, sex, food, accommodation and can be used in significant samples.

Although many mammalian species simulate human healing, none can really match it. In rat skin there is no definition between papillary dermis and reticular dermis. This animal does not form hypertrophic scars or keloids, has a thicker dermis and no subcutaneous fatty tissue or subcutaneous muscle tissue. The blood vessels are subdermal and have the same macro and microvascularisation perfusion changes (SANTOS, 2006; BETTES, 2003).

In this study, monopolar radiofrequency was chosen because it has positive results in the treatment of sagging skin, an increase in fibroblasts and collagen, which have a major influence on healing.

However, the radiofrequency device was developed for use on humans, and the size of its application handle and especially the size of the current-carrying plate are relevant factors that may have influenced the results. The fact that the handle was not completely in contact with the rat's skin and that some of the animals urinated during the application of the radiofrequency while anaesthetised was a determining factor in the episode of burns on the rat's skin, which suggests that in future studies some way should be found of emptying the bladder of these animals before the procedure.

When comparing the GC7 and GR7 groups in relation to evaluations of wound contraction at the time of surgery, day 1, day 3 and euthanasia, a significantly smaller area was found on day 3 in the GC7 compared to the GR7 ($p=0.009$). When comparing the area on the day of euthanasia of GC14 and GR14, a smaller area was found in GC14 in relation to GR14, showing a significant difference of ($p=0.001$), showing that macroscopically in the healing of cutaneous wounds, radiofrequency prolonged the inflammatory process by reducing wound contraction in the groups in which radiofrequency was applied.

In the macroscopic analysis of the punch, in which it was observed whether or not there was re-epithelialisation of the wound, in GC7, 30% were re-epithelialised while only 8.34% closed in GR7, 90.91% of the wounds in GC14 closed, while 60% closed in GR14, showing the possible influence that radiofrequency had on the re-epithelialisation of the wounds.

Histological assessment of the healing process was carried out using haematoxylin-eosin staining as it is a simple and suitable technique for quantifying and identifying cellular elements in the inflammatory, proliferative and remodelling phases of the healing process. The inflammatory reaction is important for healing, but is a harmful factor if it is intense, as it compromises local microcirculation and fibroblast proliferation (GOMES, 2006).

Correlating wound contraction with HE, it was observed that the wound did not heal completely and remained ulcerated after radiofrequency in the GR14. On the 14th P.O., there was a higher number of inflammatory cell component cells and cellular elements of acute inflammation: neutrophils compared to the control group.

In the GR7, the number of chronic inflammation cells was reduced, presumably due to the aggressive agent, possibly radiofrequency, showing that the influence of heat causes healing attempts by replacing the damaged tissue with connective tissue (ROBBINS; COTRAN, 2010).

When comparing the CG and GR groups in relation to the HE variables (inflammation, acute inflammation, chronic inflammation, fibroblastic inflammation and repair). The findings suggest that in the GR14 the fact that radiofrequency increases vasodilation, heat and oedema increased the inflammatory process for longer.

Inflammation was similar in GC7 and GR7, which is to be expected given the repair time. On the other hand, in GC14 there was a reduction in inflammation at the 14th PO, while in GR14 the inflammatory process persisted. These findings suggest that radiofrequency increases vasodilation, heat and oedema, thus increasing the inflammatory process for longer and impairing repair. The authors Borges (2010) and Carvalho (2011) state that due to the action of chemotactic agents, the inflammatory phase ends after seven days, although an increase in vessels is noted in the region.

Chronic inflammation was present in GC14 and GR14, similar to the literature, given that chronic inflammation has a prolonged duration and can last for weeks or months (ROBBINS; COTRAN 2010).

In the results, an increase in acute inflammation cells was found in GR14, which according to Robbins & Cotran (2010), should not occur in this phase, as acute inflammation is a response that serves to bring leukocytes and plasma proteins to the injured site. Since inflammation only ends when the offending agent is eliminated, these findings suggest that the influence of radiofrequency in this group was to prolong the inflammatory process. The inflammatory response is linked to the repair process; at the same time as it destroys, dilutes and removes the injurious agents, it tries to repair the damaged tissue. Repair begins during inflammation, but usually ends after the injurious influence, which in this case may have been caused by radiofrequency, has ceased.

In the study by Choi et al (2012) in which radiofrequency sessions were carried out on rabbits, histological analysis found more prominent inflammatory reactions with intense inflammatory cell growth associated with acute inflammation when compared to the control group. This effect became more prominent with evolution, showing nanostructural changes in dermal collagen fibrils.

According to the results of the study by Carvalho et al (2011), which analysed the effects of applying 3 radiofrequency sessions every other day to the skin of 20 rats, seven days after the applications the collagen underwent changes, becoming denser, with the presence of neocollagenesis. After 15 days, there was no more significant neocollagen formation, but neoelastogenesis was present on the 15th and 21st days. An intense inflammatory process was observed with the presence of epithelial shedding and oedematous areas 24 hours after RF application. These results are similar to those of Brown and Almeida (2005), suggesting that RF generates inflammation in the tissue where it was applied, with the formation of oedema, increased vascularisation and blood flow, which can generate haemorrhages and the stimulation of fibroblasts. Similar findings were also found in this study.

In the studies by Carvalho et al (2011), it was possible to conclude in relation to the effects of radiofrequency on collagen tissue, that three applications using a temperature of 37 degrees for two minutes on the back of Wistar rats resulted in neocollagenesis in the analyses corresponding to sacrifices at 24 hours and 7 days after the last application. In the groups sacrificed at 15 and 21 days, it was not possible to find changes in collagen tissue or the presence of neocollagenesis. However, after investigating possible changes in elastic fibres, neoelastogenesis was found.

Similar studies have been found in the literature, but with the use of other equipment, such as the cicatricial influence of the laser on the healing of rats. Heat can alter the healing process, which is often complex and unpredictable, and can often lead to hypertrophic or keloid scars. In the study by Mordon (2010), the laser was applied immediately after the breast incision was sutured, with a fluence of $110J/cm^2$. This study showed a marked decrease in type I collagen and fibronectin in laser-treated scars, as well as a decrease in type III collagen, bearing in mind that the pathological healing process is associated with a high rate of type I and type III collagen, while a low value leads to a healing process.

According to Brown and Almeida (2005), radiofrequency causes a series of inflammatory events in the tissue, including increased vascularisation, blood flow and oedema, which can cause haemorrhages and the stimulation of fibroblasts. Corroborating Del Pino's (2006) statement, radiofrequency increases the temperature in the deeper layers of the dermis, causing morphological changes such as an increase in fibroblasts and vascularisation.

Abercrombie, Flint and James (1954 apud Yaguishita 2006) studied the contraction and physiological collagenisation of quadrangular lumbar back injuries in rats, which are the most important mechanisms of tissue repair in these animals. Contraction began on the 5th postoperative day and ended 10 days later, while fibrosis began on the 5th day and continued after contraction ended and collagen fibres appeared 25 days after the experiment.

As a result, the effects of radiofrequency on the contraction and healing process were generally poor for use in the initial post-operative period, encouraging further research to assess the formation and quantity of collagen. Prospects point to a later application of radiofrequency in the post-operative period of skin healing in order to observe the results in another phase of healing, in agreement with Agne (2009) who showed that the effects of radiofrequency remain for 1 to 4 months after application. Another recommendation is to reduce the dose of radiofrequency.

Further studies with other types of animals that are more similar to human skin tissue should be carried out, evaluating differences in radiofrequency dosimetry, temperature used, number of sessions and the number of collagen cells counted.

CHAPTER 6

CONCLUSION

With regard to the effects of radiofrequency, it can be concluded that after three applications of radiofrequency on alternate days using a temperature of 38° on the back of Wistar rats, the wounds treated with radiofrequency show:

1- Delayed contraction of excisional wounds.
2- Prolongation of the acute inflammatory process, which lasts longer than physiological, probably due to the influence of radiofrequency, keeping the wound ulcerated.

REFERENCES

ABRAHAM, M. T.; MASHKEVICH, G. Monopolar Radiofrequency SkinTightening. **Facial Plast Surg Clin N Am**, v. 15. p 169-177, 2007.

AGNE, J.E. **I know electrotherapy**. Santa Maria-RS: Editora Pallotti, 2009.

AGNE, J.E. **Electrothermophototherapy**. 1. ed. Santa Maria, RS: O Autor, 2013.

BROWN, A.; ALMEIDA, G. Novel radiofrequency device for cellulite & body reshaping therapy. **Alma Laser**, São Paulo. 2005. Available at: http://www.almalasers.com/int/. Accessed on: 30/08/2014.

ATIYEH, B.S.; DIBO, S.A. Nonsurgical nonablative treatment of aging skin: radiofrequency technologies between aggressive marketing and evidence- based efficacy. **Aesthetic Plast Surg**, v. 33, n.3, p. 283-94. May 2009.

BALBINO, C.A.; PEREIRA, L.M.; CURI, R. Mechanisms involved in healing: a review. **Rev. Bras. Cienc. Farm**, São Paulo, v. 41, n. 1, p. 27-51, jan./mar. 2005.

BETTES, P.S.L. **Comparative histological and etensiometric analysis between the healing of skin wounds treated with adhesiveoctyl-2-cyanoacrylate and intradermal suture in rats.** Thesis (Doctorate in Clinical Surgery) - Federal University of Paraná, Curitiba, 2003.

BOCK, V.; NORONHA, A.F. Stimulation of neocollagenesis through radiofrequency, **Rev**

eletrônica Saúde e Ciência. Dianópolis, v. 3, n. 2, p.7-17, 2013.

BORGES, F. S.; SCORZA, F. A.; JAHARA, R. S. **Modalidades terapêuticas nas disfunções estéticas**. São Paulo: Phortes, 2010.
BLOOM, B.S.; EMER, J.; GOLDBERG, D.J. Assessment of safety and efficacy of a bipolar fractionated radiofrequency device in the treatment of photo damaged skin.**J Cosmet Laser Ther**. New York, v.14, n. 5, p. 20811, 2012.

BRASILEIRO FILHO, G.; BOGLIOLO, L. **Basic general pathology**. 6. ed. Rio de Janeiro: Guanabara Koogan, 2000.

BRAVO, B.S.F.; ISSA, M.C.A.; MUNIZ, R.L.S.; TORRADO, C.M.
Treatment of gynoid lipodystrophy with unipolar radiofrequency: clinical, laboratory and ultrasound evaluation. **Surg Cosmet Dermatol**, Rio de Janeiro, v. 5, n. 2,p. 138-144, 2013.

CAETANO, G. F. **Chitosan-alginate biomembrane in the healing of cutaneous ulcers in rats.** Dissertation (Master's in Biotechnology)- University of São Paulo, São Paulo, 2012.

CAMARGO, P.A. **Immunohistochemical study of angiogenesis and fibrogenesis in the vocal fold of pigs after excision of a mucosal fragment using cold instruments and CO2 laser**. Thesis (Doctorate in Clinical Surgery) - Federal University of Paraná, Curitiba, 2007.

CARVALHO, G.F.; SILVA, R.M.V.; MESQUITA, J.J.T.F.; MEYER, P.F.; RONZIO, O.A.; MEDEIROS, J.O, et al. Evaluation of the effects of radiofrequency on connective tissue. **Especial Dermatologia**, Natal, RN, v. 68, 2011.

CLARK, R.A.F.; ADAM, J.; SINGER, M.D.; RICHARD, A.F. Cutaneous wound healing. **The New England Journal of Medicine,** Massachusetts, 1999.

CEPEDA, A.M.C.; ERZINGER, G.F.D. Effects of radiofrequency on abdominal fat. **Revista Inspirar Movimento & Saúde**, v. 4, n.1, p.15-21, jan./feb. 2012.
COSTA, E.M.; MEYER, P.F.; FURTADO, F.N.B.; MEDEIROS, M.L.; DANTAS, J.S.C.; RONZIO, O.A. Evaluation of the effects of the use of tecatherapy on abdominal adiposity. **K**, 2009.

CHOI, S.; CHEONG, Y.; SHIN, J.H.; LEE, H.J.; LEE, G.J.; CHOI, S.K.;
JIN, K.H.; PARK, H.K. Short-term nanostructural effects of high radiofrequency treatment on the skin tissues of rabbits. **Lasers Med Sci**, Korea, v. 27, n.5, p. 923-33. Sep 2012.

DEL PINO, E. et al. Effect of controlled volumetric tissue heating with radiofrequency on cellulite and the subcutaneous tissue of the buttocks and thighs. **J of Drugs in Dermatol**, México, v. 5, Sep 2006.

EHRLICH, H. P.; KRUMMEL, T. M. Regulation of wound healing from a connective tissue perspective. **Wound Repair Regen.**, v. 4, p. 203-6, 1996.

FITZPATRICK, R.; GERONEMUS,R.; GOLDBERG, D.;KAMINER, M.; KILMER, S.; RUIZ-ESPARZA, J. Multicenter study of noninvasive radiofrequency for periorbital tissue tightening. **Lasers Surg Med,** v. 33, n. 4, p. 232-42, 2003. Available at: http://www.ncbi.nlm.nih.gov/pubmed/14571447. Accessed on : 23/04/14

FORREST, L. Current concepts in soft connective tissue wound healing (review). **Br. J. Surg,** Guildford, v. 70, p.133-42, 1983.

GUIRRO, E.; GUIRRO,R. **Dermatofunctional Physiotherapy.** 3. ed. São Paulo: Manole, 2002.

GUIRRO, E.; GUIRRO, R. **Dermato-Functional Physiotherapy: fundamentals, resources and pathologies.** 3 ed. São Paulo: Manole, 2007.

GEDDES, L.A.; SILVA L.F.; DEWITT, D.P.; PEARCE, J.A. What's new in electrosurgical instrumentation ? **Med Instrum.** v. 11, n. 6, p. 355-61, 1977. Available at : http://www.ncbi.nlm.nih.gov/pubmed/340856 Accessed on 25/5/2014.
GOMES, C.S.; CAMPOS, A.C.L.; TORRES, O.J.M.; VASCONCELOS, P.R.L.; MOREIRA, A.T.R.; TENÓRIO, S.B.;et al.Efeito do extrato de passiflora edulis na cicatrização da parede abdominal de ratos: estudo morfológico e tensiometétrico.Acta Cirúrgica Brasileira.2006; v 21 (2).

HARTH, Y.; LISCHINSKY, D. A novel method for real-time skin impedance measurement during radiofrequency skin tightening treatments. **Journal of Cosmetic Dermatology**, New York, v. 10, p. 24-29, 2011.

HUPP, J.R.; PETTERSON, L.J.; ELLIS III, E. ; HUPP, J.R.; TUCKER, M.R. **Wound repair**. Ed Contemporary oral and maxillofacial surgery. Rio de Janeiro: Guanabara Koogan, 2000.

JUNQUEIRA, L.C.; CARNEIRO, J. **Basic Histology**. Rio de Janeiro: Guanabara Koogan, 2004.

LANGE, A. **Dermato-functional physiotherapy applied to plastic surgery**. Curitiba: Vitória Gráfica & Editor, 2014.

KITCHEN, S.; BAZIN, S. **Electrotherapy evidence-based practice.** 11. ed. São Paulo: Manole, 2003.

MANDELBAUM, S.H.; SANTIS, E.P.D.; MANDELBAUM, M.H.S. Scarring: Current concepts and auxiliary resources - Part I. **An Bras Dermatol**, Rio de Janeiro, v. 4, n. 1, p. 393-410, 2003.

MATTOS, R.; FILIPPO, A.; TOREZAN, L. CAMPOS, V. Non-laser energy sources in rejuvenation: part II. **Surgical and Cosmetic Dermatologi,** Rio de Janeiro, v. 1, n. 2, April/June 2009.

MORDON, S.; CAPON, A.; FOURNIER, N.; IARMARCOVAI, G. Lasers thermiques et cicatrisation cutanée. **Medecine/Sciences,** France, v. 26. p. 89-94. 2010.

MOREIRA, J. A. R; GIUSTI, H. H. K.D. Dermato-functional physiotherapy in the treatment of stretch marks: a literature review. **Revista Científica da Uniararas,** São Paulo, v. 1, n.2, 2013.

NASCIMENTO, D.S., NIWA, A. B. M. ;OSÓRIO, N. **Radiofrequência e infravermeho-2008.** Indexed in Lilacs Virtual under LLXP: S0034- 72642008000900004.

NARESSE, L.E.et al. Effect of faecal peritonitis on the healing of the distal colon in the rat: anatomopathological evaluation, study of rupture force and tissue hydroxyproline. **Acta Cir Bras**, v. 8, n. 2, p. 48-53.1993.

RIBEIRO, C.T. D. **Effects of hydrogel treatment on the healing of lower limb venous ulcers: a systematic review.** 2014. Dissertation (Master's in Movement and Health) - Federal University of Rio Grande do Norte, Natal, 2014.

RISPOLI, D.Z. **Intracordal corticoid: effect on vocal fold healing after mucosal fragment excision with CO laser[2] in pigs.** Dissertation (Master's Degree in Clinical Surgery) - Federal University of Paraná, Curitiba, 2006.

ROBBINS, F. R. **Structural and Functional Pathology**. 6. ed. Rio de Janeiro: Guanabara Koogan, 2001.

ROBBINS, l.; COTRAN, R. **Pathology. Pathological Basis of Diseases.** Rio de Janeiro: Elsevier, 2010.

ROCHA, J.C.T. Laser therapy, tissue healing and angiogenesis. **Ver Bras Pesq Sau,** Ceará, v. 17, n. 1, p. 44-8, 2004.

SANTOS, M. F. S.; CZECZKO, N. G.; NASSIF, P.A.N.; FILHO, J.M.R.; ALENCAR, B.L.F.; MALAFAIA, O, et al. Evaluation of the use of the crude extract of Jatropha gossypiifolia L. in the healing of cutaneous wounds in rats. **Acta Cir Bras**, v. 21, n. 3, p. 2-7, 2006. Available at URL: http://www.scielo.br/acb

SINNO, H.; MALHOTRA, M.; LUTFY J.et al. The effects of topical collagen treatment on wound breaking strength and scar cosmesis in rats. **Can J Plast Surg,** Canada, v. 20, n. 3, p. 181-185. 2012.

SIMÕES, N.P. **Comparative study between He-Ne laser and electrical stimulation in the healing process of rat skin.** Dissertation

(Master's Degree in Health Technology) Catholic University of Paraná, Curitiba, 2007.

SCHURCH, W.; SEEMAYER, T.; GABBIANI, G. The myofibroblast. A quarter century after its discovery**. Am. J. Surg. Pathol.**, New York, v. 22, n. 2, p. 141-7, 1998.

TOLAZZI, A.R.D. **Effect of the leukotriene inhibitor montelukast on skin healing in rats: tensiometric evaluation, scar contraction and collagen deposition**. Dissertation (Master's Degree in Clinical Surgery)-Federal University of Paraná, Curitiba, 2007.
Available at:
http://dspace.c3sl.ufpr.br:8080/dspace/bitstream/handle/1884/13848/EFEI T0%20D0%20M0NTELUCASTE%20NA%20CICATRIZA%c3%87%c3% 83O%20CUT%c3%82NEA%20EM%2GRATOS.pdf?sequence=1. Accessed on 02/11/2013.

VALENTE, F. S. **Topical therapy in the healing of skin lesions caused by freezing with liquid nitrogen in Wistar rats.** Dissertation (Master's Degree in Veterinary Sciences) - Federal University of Rio Grande do Sul, Porto Alegre, 2014.

YAGUISHITA, N.; **Healing induced by porous cellulose membrane (membracel) in rat dorsum.** Dissertation (Master's Degree in Clinical Surgery) - Federal University of Paraná, Curitiba, 2006.

ANNEXES

ANNEX 1

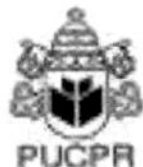

Pontifícia Universidade Católica do Paraná

Núcleo de Bioética
Comitê de Ética no Uso de Animais

Curitiba, 28 de fevereiro de 2013.

PARECER DE PROTOCOLO DE PESQUISA

REGISTRO DO PROJETO: 684 – 3ª versão

TÍTULO DO PROJETO: Efeitos da radiofrequência analisados por planigrafia e histologia na cicatrização de feridas cutâneas em ratos

PESQUISADOR RESPONSÁVEL: Ana Maria Cardoso Cepeda

EQUIPE DE PESQUISA:

Ana Maria Cardoso Cepeda

INSTITUIÇÃO:

Pontifícia Universidade Católica do Paraná

ESCOLA / CURSO:

Mestrado em clinica cirurgica

ESPÉCIE DE ANIMAL	SEXO	IDADE / PESO	CATEGORIA	QUANTIDADE
Ratos Wistar	Machos	3 meses / 300-350g	C	48

O colegiado do CEUA em reunião no dia 28/02/2013, avaliou o projeto e emite o seguinte parecer: **APROVADO.**

PUCPR de forma clara e sucinta, identificando a parte do protocolo a ser modificado e as suas justificativas.

Se houver mudança do protocolo o pesquisador deve enviar um relatório ao CEUA-PUCPR descrevendo de forma clara e sucinta, a parte do protocolo a ser modificado e as suas justificativas.

Se a pesquisa, ou parte dela for realizada em outras instituições, cabe ao pesquisador não iniciá-la antes de receber a autorização formal para a sua realização. O documento que autoriza o início da pesquisa deve ser carimbado e assinado pelo responsável da instituição e deve ser mantido em poder do pesquisador responsável, podendo ser requerido por este CEUA em qualquer tempo.

Lembramos ao pesquisador que é obrigatório encaminhar o relatório anual parcial e relatório final da pesquisa a este CEUA.

Atenciosamente,

Prof.ª Graciela Maria D'Almeida e Oliveira
Coordenadora Adjunta
Comitê de Ética no Uso de Animais

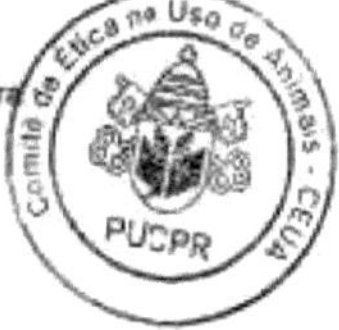

ANNEX 2

Presidency of the Republic
Civil House
Deputy Head of Legal Affairs

LAW NO. 11.794, OF 8 OCTOBER 2008.

Regulates item VII of § 1 of art. 225 of the Federal Constitution, establishing procedures for the scientific use of animals;
revokes Law No. 6.638, of 8 May 1979; and makes other provisions.

THE PRESIDENT OF THE REPUBLIC I make known that the National Congress decrees and I sanction the following Law:

CHAPTER I

PRELIMINARY PROVISIONS

Art. 1 The breeding and use of animals in teaching and scientific research activities, throughout the national territory, obeys the criteria established in this Law.

§ 1 The use of animals in educational activities is restricted to:

1 - higher education establishments;

11 - establishments of technical professional education at secondary level in the biomedical area.

20 2 Scientific research activities are all those related to basic science, applied science, technological development, production and quality control of drugs, medicines, foodstuffs, immunobiologicals, instruments or any other tested on animals, as defined in specific regulations.

§ 30 Zootechnical practices related to farming are not considered research activities.

Art. 2 The provisions of this Law apply to animals of the species classified as phylum **Chordata**, subphylum **Vertebrata,** subject to environmental legislation.

Art. 3 For the purposes of this Law, the following definitions shall apply:

I - phylum **Chordata**: animals whose exclusive characteristics, at least in the embryonic stage, are the presence of a notochord, gill slits in the pharynx and a single dorsal nerve tube;

II - **Vertebrate** subphylum: chordate animals whose exclusive characteristics are a large encephalon enclosed in a cranial box and a vertebral column;

III - experiments: procedures carried out on live animals to elucidate physiological or pathological phenomena using specific, pre-established techniques;

IV - death by humane means: the killing of an animal under conditions that involve, depending on the species, a minimum of physical or mental suffering.

Sole Paragraph. An experiment is not considered an experiment:

I - the prophylaxis and veterinary treatment of the animal that needs it;

II - the ringing, tattooing, marking or application of another method for the purpose of identifying the animal, provided that it causes only momentary pain or distress or temporary damage;

III - non-experimental interventions related to agricultural practices.

CHAPTER II

OF THE NATIONAL COUNCIL FOR THE CONTROL OF ANIMAL EXPERIMENTATION - CONCEA

Art. 4 The National Council for the Control of Animal Experimentation (CONCEA) is hereby created.

Art. 5 CONCEA is responsible for:

IV- formulating and ensuring compliance with the rules on the humane use of animals for teaching and scientific research purposes;

V I - accredit institutions for the breeding or use of animals in teaching and scientific research;

VI I - monitor and evaluate the introduction of alternative techniques that replace the use of animals in teaching and research;

VII - establish and periodically review the standards for the use and care of animals for teaching and research, in line with the international conventions to which Brazil is a signatory;

VIII - establishing and periodically reviewing technical standards for the installation and operation of breeding centres, vivariums and animal experimentation laboratories, as well as working conditions in such facilities;

IX - establishing and periodically reviewing standards for the accreditation of institutions that breed or use animals for teaching and research;

X II - to keep an up-to-date record of teaching and research procedures carried out or in progress in the country, as well as researchers, based on information sent by the Ethics Committees on the Use of Animals - CEUAs, referred to in Article 8 of this Law;

XI II - to assess and decide on appeals against CEUA decisions;

XII - draw up and submit its internal regulations to the Minister of State for Science and Technology for approval;

XIII - advise the executive branch on the teaching and research activities covered by this law.

Art. 6 CONCEA is made up of:

I - Plenary;

II - Permanent and Temporary Chambers;

III - Executive Secretariat.

§ 10 CONCEA's Permanent and Temporary Chambers will be defined in the internal regulations.

§ 20 The Executive Secretariat is responsible for CONCEA's office and will have the administrative support of the Ministry of Science and Technology.

§ 30 CONCEA may make use of **ad hoc** consultants of recognised technical and scientific competence to instruct any processes on its agenda.

Art. 7 CONCEA will be chaired by the Minister of State for Science and Technology and made up of:

1 - 1 (one) representative from each of the following bodies and organisations:

a) Ministry of Science and Technology;

b) National Council for Scientific and Technological Development - CNPq;

c) Ministry of Education;

d) Ministry of the Environment;

e) Ministry of Health;

f) Ministry of Agriculture, Livestock and Supply;

g) Council of Rectors of the Universities of Brazil - CRUB;

h) Brazilian Academy of Sciences;

i) Brazilian Society for the Advancement of Science;

j) Federation of Experimental Biology Societies;

l) Brazilian College of Animal Experimentation;

m) National Federation of the Pharmaceutical Industry;

II - 2 (two) representatives of animal protection societies legally established in the country.

§ Paragraph 1 In the event that the Minister of State for Science and Technology is prevented from attending, he shall be replaced as CONCEA President by the Executive Secretary of the respective Ministry.

§ The President of CONCEA shall have the casting vote.

§ Paragraph 3 CONCEA members shall not be remunerated, and the services they provide shall be considered, for all intents and purposes, a relevant public service.

CHAPTER III

of the ethics committees for the use of animals - CEUAs

Art. 8 It is an indispensable condition for the accreditation of institutions that carry out teaching or research activities with animals to set up Ethics Committees for the Use of Animals - CEUAs.

Art. 9 CEUAs are made up of:

§ 1 veterinarians and biologists;

§ 11 teachers and researchers in the specific field;

§ 111 - 1 (one) representative of animal protection societies legally established in the country, in accordance with the Regulations.

Art. 10. The CEUAs are responsible for:

§ 112 to comply with and enforce, within the scope of their duties, the provisions of this Law and other rules applicable to the use of animals for teaching and research, especially CONCEA resolutions;

§ 113examine in advance the teaching and research procedures to be carried out at the institution to which it is linked, to determine their compatibility with the applicable legislation;

§ 114 - keep an up-to-date record of teaching and research procedures carried out or in progress at the institution, sending a copy to CONCEA;

§ 115 maintain a register of researchers who carry out teaching and research procedures, sending a copy to CONCEA;

§ 116issue, within the scope of their duties, certificates that may be required by research funding bodies, scientific journals or others;

§ 117 Immediately notify CONCEA and the health authorities of any accidents involving animals in accredited institutions, providing information to enable remedial action to be taken.

§ 118 If any procedure is found to be in breach of the provisions of this Law in the execution of a teaching or research activity, the respective CEUA will order its execution to be paralysed until the irregularity is remedied, without prejudice to the application of other applicable sanctions.

§ 119 In the event of the hypothesis set out in § 1 of this article, the CEUA's failure to act will result in sanctions for the institution, under the terms of arts. 17 and 20 of this Law.

§ 120 Decisions handed down by the CEUAs can be appealed, without suspensive effect, to CONCEA.

§ 121 The members of the CEUAs will be held responsible for any damage that they cause to ongoing research through wilful misconduct.

§ 122 The members of the CEUAs are obliged to protect industrial secrets, under penalty of liability.

CHAPTER IV

CONDITIONS FOR THE BREEDING AND USE OF ANIMALS FOR TEACHING AND LEARNING

SCIENTIFIC RESEARCH

Art. 11: It is the responsibility of the Ministry of Science and Technology to licence the animal breeding, teaching and scientific research activities referred to in this Law.

§ Paragraph 1 (VETOED)

§ Paragraph 2 (VETOED)

§Paragraph 3 (VETOED)

Art. 12: The breeding or use of animals for research is restricted exclusively to institutions accredited by CONCEA.

Art. 13: Any institution legally established in the country that breeds or uses animals for teaching and research must apply to CONCEA for accreditation for the use of animals, provided that it has previously set up a CEUA.

§ 10 At the discretion of the institution and with the authorisation of CONCEA, the creation of more than one CEUA per institution is permitted.

§ 20 In the case provided for in § 1 of this article, each CEUA will define the animal experimentation laboratories, animal houses and breeding centres under its control.

Art. 14: The animal can only be subjected to the interventions recommended in the protocols of the experiments that make up the research or learning programme when, before, during and after the experiment, it receives special care, as established by CONCEA.

§ 21 The animal will be euthanised, in strict compliance with the relevant prescriptions for each species, according to the guidelines of the Ministry of Science and Technology, whenever the experiment or any of its phases is technically recommended or when intense suffering occurs.

§ 22 Exceptionally, when the animals used in experiments or demonstrations are not to be euthanised, they may leave the vivarium after the intervention, after consulting the respective CEUA regarding current safety criteria, provided that they are sent to suitable people or duly legalised animal protection organisations who wish to take responsibility for them.

§ 30 Whenever possible, teaching practices should be photographed, filmed or recorded so that they can be reproduced to illustrate future practices, avoiding unnecessary repetition of teaching procedures with animals.

§ 40 The number of animals to be used for a project and the duration of each experiment will be the minimum necessary to produce a conclusive result, sparing the animal as much suffering as possible.

§ 50 Experiments that may cause pain or distress will be carried out under appropriate sedation, analgesia or anaesthesia.

§ 60 Experiments aimed at studying processes related to pain and anguish require specific authorisation from CEUA, in compliance with the rules established by CONCEA.

§ 70 The use of neuromuscular blockers or muscle relaxants as a substitute for sedative, analgesic or anaesthetic substances is prohibited.

§ 80 It is forbidden to reuse the same animal once the main objective of the research project has been achieved.

§ 90 In a teaching programme, whenever traumatic procedures are used, several procedures can be carried out on the same animal, as long as they are all carried out under a single anaesthetic and the animal is sacrificed before it regains consciousness.

§ 10 In order to carry out animal breeding and experimentation work in closed systems, the safety conditions and standards recommended by the international organisations to which Brazil is bound will be taken into account.

Art. 15 - CONCEA, taking into account the relationship between the level of suffering for the animal and the practical results expected to be obtained, may restrict or prohibit experiments that involve a high degree of aggression.

Art. 16: Every scientific research project or teaching activity will be supervised by a graduate or post-graduate professional in the biomedical field, linked to a teaching or research organisation accredited by CONCEA.

CHAPTER V

PENALTIES

Art. 17: Institutions that carry out activities regulated by this Law are subject, in the event of transgression of its provisions and regulations, to the administrative penalties of:

I - warning;

II - a fine of between R$ 5,000.00 (five thousand reais) and R$ 20,000.00 (twenty thousand reais);

III - temporary ban;

IV - suspension of funding from official sources of credit and scientific development;

V - permanent ban.

Sole Paragraph. A ban of more than 30 (thirty) days can only be determined by an act of the Minister of State for Science and Technology, after hearing CONCEA.

Art. 18 Any person who improperly carries out activities regulated by this Law or participates in procedures not authorised by CONCEA shall be liable to the following administrative penalties:

I - warning;

II - a fine of between R$ 1,000.00 (one thousand reais) and R$ 5,000.00 (five thousand reais);

III - temporary suspension;

IV - a definitive ban on the exercise of the activity regulated in this Law.

The penalties provided for in articles 17 and 18 of this Law will be applied according to the seriousness of the offence, the damage caused by it, the aggravating or mitigating circumstances and the offender's background.

The sanctions provided for in articles 17 and 18 of this Law shall be applied by CONCEA, without prejudice to the corresponding criminal liability.

Art. 21: Supervision of the activities regulated by this law is the responsibility of the bodies of the Ministries of Agriculture, Livestock and Supply, Health, Education, Science and Technology and the Environment, in their respective areas of competence.

CHAPTER VI

GENERAL AND TRANSITIONAL PROVISIONS

Art. 22: Institutions that breed or use animals for teaching or research that existed in the country before the effective date of this Law must:

I - create the CEUA within a maximum of 90 (ninety) days of the regulations referred to in Article 25 of this Law;

II - make their physical facilities compatible, within a maximum period of 5 (five) years from the entry into force of the rules established by CONCEA, based on item V of the **caput of** Article 5 of this Law.

Art. 23 CONCEA, by means of a resolution, will recommend to scientific research funding agencies that projects be rejected for any of the following reasons:

I - that are being carried out without CEUA approval;

II - whose realisation has been suspended by CEUA.

Art. 24: The budgetary resources necessary for CONCEA to function will be provided for in the appropriations of the Ministry of Science and Technology.

Art. 25: This law will be regulated within 180 (one hundred and eighty) days.

Art. 26 This Law shall enter into force on the date of its publication.

Art. 27. Law no.º 6.638, of 8 May 1979, is hereby repealed.

Brasília, 8th October 2008; 187º da Independência e 120º da República.

LUIZ INÁCIO LULA DA SILVA
Tarso Genro
Reinhold Stephanes
José Gomes Temporão
Miguel Jorge
Luiz Antonio Rodrigues Elias
Carlos Minc

ANNEX 3

Analysing HE

CASE	INFLAMMATION	CHRONIC INFLAMMATION	INFLAMMATION WATCH OUT	FIBROBLAST PROLIFERATION	REPAIR	RE-EPITHELIALISATION OBS
1Q7	3	2	4	3	2-	
2Q14	3	3	2	3	1-	
2P14	2	2	0	2	1+	
4P14	3	2	3	2	1-	
4Q14	4	2	4	2	3-	
10P14	2	1	1	3	1-	
10Q14	4	2	4	3	1-	
11P14	1	2	0	2	4+	
11Q14	3	2	3	3	1-	
13Q14C	3	2	1	3	4-	
13P14C	2	2	0	2	3+	
15P7C	3	3	1	3	4-	
16P14C	1	1	0	2	1+	
16Q14C	2	2	1	3	1-	
17P14C	1	1	0	2	2+	
17Q14C	3	2	3	2	2-	
18P7C	2	2	2	2	1-	
18Q7C	3	3	2	3	1-	
19P14C	1	1	0	2	1+	
19Q14C	2	2	2	3	1-	
20P14C	1	1	0	2	1+	
24P7C	2	2	1	2	1-	
24Q7C	3	2	2	3	1-	
27Q7	3	3	2	3	1-	
29P14	1	1	0	2	1+	
29Q14	2	1	4	1	1-	
31P14	1	1	0	2	1+	
31Q14	3	1	4	1	1-	NECROSE
32P14	1	1	0	2	2+	
32Q14	3	2	2	3	1-	
33P14	2	2	1	2	3-	
33Q14	4	2	4	2	1-	NECROSE
36P14	2	2	1	2	1-	
36Q14	3	2	3	3	2-	
37P14C	1	1	0	2	2+	
37Q14C	3	2	1	3	4-	
38P7C	2	2	2	2	3+	
38Q7C	3	2	3	3	2-	
39Q7C	2	3	2	3	2-	
39P7C	2	1	2	2	1-	
43Q14C	2	3	0	2	4+	

43P14C	2	2	1	2	4-
41P7C	2	2	1	3	1-
41Q7C	3	3	2	3	1-
42Q7C	3	2	2	2	1-
42P7C	1	1	0	2	1-
44Q7C	2	2	1	3	3-
44P7C	1	1	0	2	1+
45P7C	2	2	1	2	1-
45Q7C	3	2	2	3	1-
46Q14C	2	2	0	2	3-
46P14C	2	2	3	2	3+
50P14	1	1	0	2	1+
50Q14	3	2	2	3	1-
61P7	1	1	0	3	3+
70Q7	2	1	2	3	1-
20Q14C	2	2	2	3	1-
21P14C	1	1	0	2	2+
21Q14C	2	2	2	2	1-
22P14C	1	1	0	2	3+
22Q14C	3	3	2	2	2-
23P14C	1	1	0	2	1+
23Q14C	2	2	2	3	3-
47P7	2	2	1	3	1-
57Q7	3	2	3	3	1-
1P7	2	2	1	3	3-
15Q7C	3	3	2	3	1-
27P7	2	2	1	3	1-
57P7	2	2	1	3	3-
14P7C	2	2	1	3	1-
5Q7	3	1	4	2	1-
28P7	3	3	1	2	2+
14Q7C	3	3	2	3	2-
28Q7	2	2	1	3	1-
70P7	2	2	1	3	1-
40P7	2	2	2	2	3+
40Q7	3	2	3	3	2-
47Q7	3	3	3	2	4-
8P7	2	2	1	3	1-
26Q7	3	2	4	3	1-
61Q7	2	1	1	2	3-
26P7	1	1	1	2	2-
8Q7	2	2	1	3	1-
5P7	1	1	1	2	2-
35Q7	3	2	3	3	1-
35P7	1	1	1	3	3-

	cellular inflammatory component	
0	absence of cellular elements	
1	inflammatory cells in small numbers (near vessels)	
2	inflammatory cells in moderate numbers, sparse	
3	inflammatory cells in moderate numbers, clusters	
4	numerous inflammatory cells	

	cellular elements of chronic infection: lymphocytes	

0	absence of lymphocytes or plasma cells	
1	small number of lymphocytes and/or plasma cells	
2	moderate number of lymphocytes and/or plasma cells	
3	numerous lymphocytes/ plasma cells	
4	numerous lymphocytes, lymphoid nodules, lymphocyte crowns	

	cellular elements of acute infection: neutrophils
0	absence of neutrophils, capillary congestion
1	small number of neutrophils in the dermis
2	moderate number of neutrophils
3	exudatoneutrophilic
4	exudatoneutrophilic, abscesses

	repair: macrophages, granulomas
0	no evidence of repair
1	macrophages in small numbers
2	macrophages in moderate quantity
3	macrophages in numer.mod, without specific arrangement
4	macrophages arranged in granulomas.

	Fibroblast proliferation
0	young fibroblasts are not observed
1	fibroblasts are seen in areas of loose collagen
2	fibroblasts are easily observed, collagen matrix visible
3	easily observed fibroblasts, collagen matrix and capillary proliferation
4	fibroblasts are numerous, collagen matrix present, capillary proliferation

ANNEX 4

The areas were analysed using ImageJ® *software (National Institutes of Health*, USA) of all the rats in the two groups on the day of surgery, day 1, day 3 and euthanasia.

GROUPS	RAT NO.	AREA CX	AREA 1 DAY	AREA 3 DAY	AREA EUTHANASIA
GC 7	18	384.354	291.295	248.765	170.135
GC7	44	390.050	487.126	287.690	384.423

GC7	39	447.074	412.123	306.257	357.284
GC7	38	394.309	429.873	259.673	290.603
GC7	41	383.169	448.402	245.320	309.332
GC7	24	397.937	337.133	206.530	199.925
GC7	45	407.727	431.329	213.048	235.412
GC7	42	331.481	331.820	279.531	243.668
GC7	14	477.429	455.257	266.256	235.165
GC7	15	322.965	249.442	153.308	170.797
GR7	47	487.685	430.757	388.228	317.102
GR7	57	433.498	429.820	331.874	285.544
GR7	61	404.821	547.225	367.169	309.830
GR7	70	402.963	362.593	278.615	302.720
GR7	1	470.396	352.437	442.181	307.608
GR7	5	387.932	440.246	476.960	310.339
GR7	8	445.451	450.866	258.799	301.565
GR7	27	330.784	262.618	272.434	214.387
GR7	26	328.848	313.340	303.296	190.806
GR7	28	397.254	400.957	343.601	358.184
GR7	35	381.821	304.990	241.638	171.035
GR7	40	448.096	450.264	272.708	301.012
GC14	20	395.047	410.396	269.143	73.665
GC14	22	400.986	438.712	264.472	144.418
CG14	21	367.512	412.984	206.550	135.394
CG14	16	386.435	420.756	267.213	91.385
CG14	19	411.606	411.941	263.830	93.256
CG14	13	337.188	458.432	260.079	144.028
CG14	23	361.536	454.209	383.423	107.213
CG14	46	402.958	428.568	285.548	69.871
CG14	43	357.830	433.001	299.164	64.623
CG14	17	238.193	460.712	337.449	150.093
CG14	37	487.466	451.053	361.272	111.447
CR14	36	371.475	357.311	207.401	110.425
CR14	4	425.112	404.792	205.058	145.919
CR14	50	424.869	454.536	307.507	258.531
CR14	11	429.083	453.742	297.971	252.903
CR14	29	347.619	459.123	224.778	248.604
CR14	10	368.849	463.684	191.025	175.698
CR14	31	366.122	385.769	222.215	237.706
CR14	32	438.844	446.620	303.406	125.732
CR14	2	475.721	464.059	364.723	155.986
CR14	33	432.614	449.231	302.856	193.806

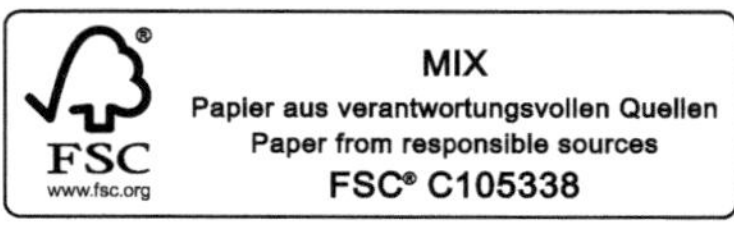

Printed by Books on Demand GmbH, Norderstedt / Germany